MW01252673

# A Bump in the Road

Thank-you for your support,
Susan

# A Bump in the Road

✦

## One Family's Journey with Cancer

*Susan L. Arnold*

*With Contributions by Brandon T. Arnold*

iUniverse, Inc.

New York  Lincoln  Shanghai

# A Bump in the Road
## One Family's Journey with Cancer

Copyright © 2007 by Susan L. Arnold

iUniverse books may be ordered through booksellers or by contacting:

iUniverse
2021 Pine Lake Road, Suite 100
Lincoln, NE 68512
www.iuniverse.com
1-800-Authors (1-800-288-4677)

Because of the dynamic nature of the Internet, any Web addresses or links contained in this book may have changed since publication and may no longer be valid.

The views expressed in this work are solely those of the author and do not necessarily reflect the views of the publisher, and the publisher hereby disclaims any responsibility for them.

ISBN: 978-0-595-46040-3 (pbk)
ISBN: 978-0-595-90340-5 (ebk)

Printed in the United States of America

*For my Family,*
*You are my strength and my joy.*

# Contents

# *Preface*

***Just*** saying the word "Cancer" evokes tremendous fear and mind numbing reactions. For a cancer patient there are shelves of books in bookstores, in libraries and in doctor's offices giving helpful tips and advice for living with the disease before, during and after treatment. There are books discussing the fear of dying, how to prepare and practical advice about financial and legal matters but rarely do the families find any material directed to them.

While family members do not actually have cancer; they are living with a serious, potentially life threatening and life altering disease which will effect everyone in some way. There is an entire spectrum of emotions and fears which family members must work through. Sometimes, just knowing what others have gone through gives our feelings validation. Although each family's experience is different it may help to know how another family coped with a similar situation.

I hope the story of my family's journey will give another family some strength, comfort and guidance as they navigate the bump in their road.

# *Acknowledgments*

*We* make the journey through life with many others who travel with us for a time and provide us with support, guidance and strength. My own journey has been filled with such special individuals and, while I couldn't begin to name all of them, those who helped me during my father's illness and the writing of this book require a tremendous public thank you for all your efforts.

In particular I'd like to thank my sons, Greg and Brandon, for their patience and willingness to take on new responsibilities because they knew I was counting on them. To my brother-in-law, Steven Arnold, who gave up a month of sleeping in his own bed to make sure our boys were awake and ready for school each morning.

To my Dad, whose bravery in the face of this disease has changed my way of thinking about living and dying and has helped reaffirm my faith. Mom, your strength and bravery has always made me proud, but never more so then now. Despite your own sorrow you still found a way to comfort a family. To my sisters, Cathy and Gail, for recognizing the added obstacles associated with my living at a distance and for finding ways to help me cope with these obstacles even while you were struggling with your own emotions and fears. To their families, Steve, Lindsay, Bradley and Rob, for the countless ways you bolstered our spirits and made this time together so meaningful. And finally, to our entire family for pulling together as a family and proving we can do anything! Dad would be so proud.

To Patty Thoma and so many others who remembered us in their prayers and took care of the little things so we didn't have to. Thank you.

And most especially, to my husband, Ron, who was, at times, the only strength I had. Who always seems to be able to read my heart and know what I need, sometimes before I know myself, and who helped care for my dad with such love and tenderness. From the bottom of my heart; thank you.

# *Introduction*

*2005* started out with such high hopes for all of us. Our family was planning a trip to Panama, Central America in February and everything in our lives seemed to be going smoothly. Everyone seemed healthy and happy. Careers were progressing well and children were growing up and becoming kind, thoughtful people. There didn't seem to be any dark clouds on the horizon. Mom and Dad had even commented about this fact and felt it was almost time for a bump in the road. We, as a family, had been very blessed and we never took these good times for granted, which is why Mom and Dad believed there is always a bump in the road to keep us humble.

The bump was rather larger than expected. Dad was diagnosed with lung cancer in April. This book is adapted from my personal journal that I kept from the day I was given the awful news. It describes the feelings of shock, numbness, denial and the never ending roller coaster of emotions which seemed to grip all of us, except Dad, who remained calm throughout it all.

As I reread this journal following Dad's passing, I realized it dealt with many practical points which are seldom talked about or forgotten and solutions to problems which can crop up. With the encouragement of my sister, Gail, my Mom and my friend, Patty, I have chosen to release my words and feelings to the world in the hope that it may, in some small way, give strength to another family and let them know others have gone through this event and survived. This is not a "how to" manual. It is a journal that shows a family's love and that wonderful moments were possible even while we were saying good-bye.

Because it is a journal it is divided into daily entries with the inclusion of e-mail messages from various family members but most often between my father and me. Also, our youngest son, Brandon, who, like me, expresses himself by writing, has contributed several entries of his own which gives us insight into the thoughts and feelings of the younger generation when a family is faced with a person dying of cancer.

If nothing else, this journal has given me the chance to re-examine those dark days and found there was more beauty then I had realized; more love and strength in each of us then we had believed and more lessons to be learned from a father whose family always came first. I also learned life's journey contains many bumps in the road. Each one will toss us around for a time and temporarily disorient us but, once we are able to examine and see the bump through the rearview mirror we will discover the bump added more to our journey then a smooth, straight highway ever could.

# *The Clark Family Tree*

### *(By Generation)*

## First Generation

Harold E. Clark and Ethel I. Clark. Retired. Lives in Sharbot Lake, Ontario

## Second Generation—Harold and Ethel's Children

| | |
|---|---|
| Susan. | Married to Ron Arnold. Municipal Treasurer. Ron owns a convenience store. They live in South River. |
| Cathy. | Married to Steve Fox. Registered Nurse. Steve works for Canadian Pacific Railway. They live in Sharbot Lake, Ontario. |
| Gail. | Companion to Rob Harding. Both work for the Ontario Ministry of Health. Gail lives in Kingston, Ontario. Rob lives in Amherstview, Ontario (near Kingston). |

## Third Generation—Harold and Ethel's Grandchildren

Lindsay Fox. Daughter of Cathy and Steve Fox. 18 years-old. Sister to Bradley Fox.

Bradley Fox. Son of Cathy and Steve Fox. 16 years-old. Brother to Lindsay Fox.

Greg Arnold. Son of Susan and Ron Arnold. 14 years-old. Brother to Brandon Arnold.

Brandon Arnold. Son of Susan and Ron Arnold. 12 years-old. Brother to Greg Arnold.

# The Arnold Family Tree

### *(By Generation)*

## First Generation

Allie and Velma (d.2000) Arnold. Retired. South River, Ontario

## Second Generation—Allie and Velma's Children

| | |
|---|---|
| Steve Arnold. | Retired. Married to Dawn. Live in South River, Ontario |
| Ron Arnold: | Store Owner. Married to Susan Clark. Lives in South River, Ontario |
| Perry Arnold: | Works for Kent Trusses. Married to Brenda. Lives in South River, Ontario |

## Third Generation—Allie and Velma's Grandchildren

Cara Arnold. Daughter of Steve and Dawn.

Melody Arnold. Daughter of Steve and Dawn.

Ryan Arnold. Son of Perry and Brenda.

Chad Arnold. Son of Perry and Brenda.

Cassandra Arnold. Daughter of Perry and Brenda.

Riley Arnold. Daughter of Perry Arnold.

Greg Arnold. Son of Ron and Susan Arnold.

Brandon Arnold. Son of Ron and Susan Arnold.

# *Geography*

**Sharbot Lake, Ontario, Canada**—Located at the intersection of Highway #7 and County Rd #38 approximately 120 km west of Ottawa, Ontario (The National Capital). The Village of Sharbot Lake is located along the shores of the lake by the same name and has long been an excellent fishing and tourist region.

Sharbot Lake is home to Harold and Ethel Clark as well as Cathy and Steve Fox.

**Kingston, Ontario, Canada**—Located on the north shore of Lake Ontario at the mouth of the St. Lawrence River. Kingston is 70 km south of Sharbot Lake via County Rd #38.

Kingston is home to Gail Clark.

**Toronto, Ontario, Canada**—Located on the north shore of Lake Ontario and is approximately 200 km west of Sharbot Lake via Highway #7. Toronto is the Provincial Capital.

**South River, Ontario, Canada**—Located on Hwy 11, approximately 65 km south of North Bay and 398 km north of Toronto and 350 km north-west of Sharbot Lake. South River has a permanent population of about 1,100 which doubles in summer.

South River is home to Susan and Ron Arnold as well as the extended Arnold family.

**Eagle Lake, South River, Ontario**—Ron and Susan Arnold's cottage and the Arnold family cottage are built on the shores of Eagle Lake in Machar Township. The lake is approximately 16 km west of South River Village. Although the two cottages are not built next door they are within walking distance from each other.

**Perth, Ontario, Canada**—Located on Highway #7 Perth, Ontario is 50 km east of SharbotLake and is home to many of Ethel Clark's sisters and their families.

**Arden, Ontario, Canada**—The small village of Arden, Ontario is located 40 km west of Sharbot Lake just off Highway #7. The Clark farm, the original homestead, was established at the end of Clark Rd several kilometers south of Arden village.

# Part One

# Winter 2005

## Monday, February 28, 2005

*The* week of vacation had been wonderful. Our entire family had journeyed to Panama, Central America for what had become our annual winter holiday. We jokingly said we travelled in a pack but there was more truth in the joke than fiction! Dad and Mom have travelled every winter for the past twenty-five years. They enjoyed breaking up the cold months of winter with a week of warm, tropical sunshine. Sometimes they went on their own and other times they went with Mom's brother and his wife but always they would say how much they wished the "kids" could be with them.

When we were children Dad and Mom wanted us to see the world outside the small village we called home. They had purchased a sixteen-foot travel trailer and we pulled our home-away-from-home to some remarkable places. The five of us were able to visit Expo '67 in Montreal, Quebec and stayed in a trailer camp just outside the city. We became familiar with road signs and facilities in several provinces and northern states. Always, wherever we went, we learned about the history of the place and where it was located on a map. We would learn what a place was famous for and would visit factories, botanical gardens and attractions. What we had learned in history and geography class became real and took on a special meaning when we saw the world for ourselves. Travel was an education and Dad was a huge supporter of learning, in all its forms, all his life.

In 1998 we took our first major family holiday and headed to Disneyland in Florida. At the time, my sister Cathy's two children were eight and ten and our two boys were five and seven. They were just the right age to meet Mickey Mouse and Donald Duck in person! This was the beginning of many family holidays to distant hot spots.

We had all agreed this trip would likely be the last trip the entire family would be able to go on. Lindsay, my niece, would be heading off to university the next year and it was getting harder to arrange the schedules of twelve very busy people. We were sitting in the airport lounge in Panama and most of us were deep in our own thoughts. We were sorry the week was over and mentally beginning to prepare to re-enter the real world. Passengers were being loaded according to row numbers and when Mom and Dad's row was called they got up from their chairs and prepared to follow the crowd. Dad turned, gave us that mischievous smile he had, said they'd see us in Toronto and walked away. I remember thinking what a handsome pair they made. Dad, a young-looking seventy-three year old, was a few inches taller than Mom, his posture was so straight and he held his head high with confidence. They were both dressed casually in wind-suits, which they preferred for travelling, and their carry-on bag was slung over Dad's right shoulder. Harold and Ethel Clark was a distinguished looking couple and as they walked toward the departure gate they drew admiring glances from other travellers in the lounge.

Soon the rest of the plane was boarded and as the giant bird began to careen down the tarmac I felt my throat fill with emotion and tears spilled down my cheeks. Our youngest son, Brandon, who was twelve, turned to ask me something and saw my tears. "Are you crying, Mom?" he asked in surprise. "Yes, Honey, I'm just sad our holiday is over. I'm OK." Really, I wasn't OK. I never cry when I leave someplace. As I watched the palm trees drop away from our window I had such an overwhelming feeling that something very special was ending and for several minutes I felt a deep sense of lost and I quickly reasoned it was only because we had said, so many times on this trip, that it would be the last one with the entire family.

*Brandon*

*When I think of my Grandpa Clark I think of the great fun and adventures we've had together along with the rest of the family or just the two of us. The many trips we've taken by car, boat or even plane are imbedded in my head and, more importantly, in my heart. Grandpa was interested in everything and always wondered who, what, when, where and why. Watching him become curious made me interested too.*

*Whenever we flew somewhere Grandpa always wanted to know the name of the pilot, how big the engine was, who made it, how high up we were flying and how fast we were moving. Learning was Grandpa's hobby; like hockey is my hobby.*

*My Grandpa was a kind man. He could always find ways to help people help themselves. He respected other people's pride and opinions even if he didn't agree with them.*

*His last Christmas, December 2004, he heard about someone whose wife and children had moved out just a week before. Grandpa invited him to his house to have dinner with our family. He even made sure there were a couple presents under the tree with the man's name on them.*

*Grandpa liked toys. Maybe that's because when he was little he didn't have many. One year for Christmas I received a K'NEX set. Grandpa had dumped them all out on the floor before I even knew what they were. We spent all morning building all kinds of trucks, tractors and anything with wheels.*

*There are lots of things I miss about him. Like his giant smile, the way he could wiggle his ears, his laugh, hearing him call people "Gom" even though we have no idea what it really means and, when we would visit, waking up and going downstairs to see him at the far end of the table reading the paper with his coffee and daily orange.*

# *Part Two*

# *Spring 2005*

## Tuesday, April 26, 2005

My youngest sister, Gail, called this evening from her home in Kingston, Ontario. She had finished her final university exam earlier in the day and I thought she was calling to celebrate. Gail, already a college graduate, had decided four years ago, after working almost twenty years for the Ontario provincial government and most recently in the Ministry of Health, she wanted to study for her university degree in health sciences and had begun taking night classes at Queen's University toward that goal. Now, the years of study were behind her. Although it appeared to us like an overwhelming amount of work Gail seemed to enjoy the challenge and it seemed to agree with her. She was excited about her studies and interested in her subjects. Once Gail sets her mind to something she rarely backs off and during her years of study I often admired her staying power and her energy. We chatted about the final exam and how difficult it was and I commented on how tired she sounded. I told her she needed a hot bath and a drink to help her unwind! She laughed weakly with that prescription. Following a small silence and a deep breath she began a conversation which forever changed our lives and began a family journey unlike any we had ever taken.

Dad has been bothered by a persistent cough for several months and his family doctor had sent him for a chest x-ray in March. Dad had been a smoker from a very early age and he had finally stopped smoking five years ago on January 18, 2000. Now, his colour was good, his appetite had increased making his normally trim waistline expand and his loud breathing at night seemed to have become calm and quiet. Dad had been a pipe smoker. His ever-present pipe had always been his trademark and I loved the smell of the sweet pipe-tobacco he used. From the time we started school and learned in health class about lung disease we preached to him about the harm being done to his body from smoking. Then, to finish our sermon we would ask him to stop smoking. My mother and my two sisters and I were Dad's "girls" and there was nothing he wouldn't do for us; nothing except permanently put down the pipe. He was adamant we shouldn't follow his example and he was sorry he had gotten hooked on smoking but he said he just couldn't stop and he wished we'd stop lecturing him every time he lit his pipe. I don't think I can ever remember Dad not accomplishing something he set out to do so this admission made a huge impact with my sisters and I when we were just children. Eventually, we accepted Dad was a smoker and he was going to stay a smoker. Sometimes I was angry with his decision. Sometimes I wondered about the strength of nicotine which could control a person's life who was so in control of all the other facets of his life. Then, eighteen days into the new millennium, without an announcement or fanfare, he drew his last puff on the Brigham Three Dot pipe and never touched it again. I was so proud of him! We all were! He gave up smoking!

Doctor Bell, the family physician called to tell Dad he had seen something on the x-ray and he wanted to look at it further. He had made arrangements for a series of tests. He had a bone density test yesterday. A CT Scan from the chest up has been scheduled for tomorrow at 10:30am. The second test will be a bronchoscope scheduled for 9:00 am on Thursday. His throat will be frozen with an anesthetic spray and he will be given some valium through intervenes to relax; this will help stop the cough/swallow/gag reflex. A tube will be inserted into his left lung via his throat or his nose. A tiny camera can then be inserted through the tube as well as a little instrument to biopsy lung tissue. After, they'll "rinse" the lung with a saline solution and then suction the fluid out. They may also do some "brushing" when they rinse the lung which brushes some lung tissue cells into the saline. All of these will be analyzed (camera/rinsing fluid/biopsy). Dad was told it takes about four to five days to assess. The doctors will be looking for cancer and if they still feel things are inconclusive, they can do an MRI and/or another needle biopsy. Assuming the procedure starts on time it should take about ½ to one hour and the rest of the time he will be in recovery. He'll have a sore throat and chest, and may cough up some blood for a few days. These are all normal.

The only word which registered as Gail quietly spoke to me over the phone was *cancer*! The doctors are looking for cancer in Dad's lung!

Mom and Dad have always been private and very good at protecting our feelings and shielding us from worry. This had included, in the past, minor health issues which they hadn't told us about until they were feeling better and then, not always. Sometimes they'd mention something a year or two later and we'd be taken by surprise and say, "We didn't know that!" My younger sister, Cathy, and her husband and children live in the little village of Sharbot Lake, Ontario; the same community as Mom and Dad. Gail, my youngest sister, lives in Kingston. Sharbot Lake is 75 kilometers north of Kingston. My husband and I and our two boys live in South River, just south of North Bay, Ontario and a 350 km drive from our door to my parent's door.

When I first moved to South River Cathy, Gail and I made a pact that if they ever had a reason to suspect Mom or Dad were ill they had to tell me. In my heart I knew if anything were ever seriously wrong Mom and Dad would tell me but I also knew there would be very few advance-clues. I didn't want to feel I was out of the loop just because I lived a distance away from them. Cathy is a registered nurse and had worked for the Victoria Order of Nurses for about twenty years and was now taking a break from nursing and was spending time at home. Cathy had found out by accident because of an innocent question which made her suspicious. Mom and Dad had not wanted us to know about the testing until they had the results. They knew Gail was studying for her exam and Cathy had begun taking university courses towards her nursing degree via correspondence courses and she had an exam, too, in the near future so they didn't want to upset everyone until they had all the test results and knew the next step. Mom and Dad had planned to tell us everything when the timing was right. When Cathy asked Dad if there was anything he wanted to tell her she watched Mom and Dad exchange glances and she instinctively knew something was really wrong. Dad told her what the doctors suspected and about the tests he was scheduled to have during the week. They asked her not to say anything to the rest of the family until they had more news. Their request seemed simple, their reasoning was rational but it put Cathy in a situation she didn't know how to deal with on her own. Our family has always been close. We've always gone through the good and the bad together. How could she possibly keep this to herself? That's the thing with life; it gives us the strength to do what we would never have thought we could do. Cathy did keep their secret and even managed to organize an eighteenth birthday party for her daughter, Lindsay.

Following Gail's exam and one of Dad's appointments Mom and Dad went to Gail's house and told her what the doctors were looking for. Cathy could now share her burden with Gail. They wanted Mom and Dad to tell me but Mom and Dad wanted to wait until they had more test results before making the call to me in South River. Gail and Cathy decided to keep our pact and go against Mom and Dad's wishes (although they knew Mom and Dad would understand) and give me some advanced warning. We decided to allow Dad and Mom the peace of mind of thinking they were sparing me from worry until they had all the medical facts and test results. I would be kept in the loop without Mom and Dad knowing.

Gail concluded our call by reiterating that we were still only at the investigative stage and to try not to jump too far ahead.

Dad, who has always been our measure for any man, might be very ill. He might be dying. As I hung up the phone in the kitchen fear crept slowly into my head and my heart and I realized I was gasping for air. After some minutes I was able to regain some of my composure and focus on Gail's final words, "It is still only investigative." Yet, somewhere, deep in my very core, I was struggling between believing everything would be fine and what I instinctively knew the test results would reveal.

Ron, my husband, had overheard bits and pieces of our conversation but waited in the livingroom until I was ready to confide. Greg and Brandon, our sons, were downstairs in the Rec room. In a quiet, strangled voice I explained to Ron what was happening and then walked steadily into the bathroom to throw-up.

## Wednesday, April 27, 2005

*Sleep* had a way of blending into my consciousness all night long. When I first woke-up, I had the very happy thought that my conversation with Gail last night had been a terrible nightmare. After several minutes the knot in my stomach returned with such force I knew without a doubt what was real and what wasn't.

I knew Gail and Cathy would be concerned about me and how I was coping. What could I tell them? I couldn't even actually think the words let alone give them a voice. Yet, I felt I had to communicate to them how I was reacting. Again I was stuck; how was I reacting? I felt sick to my stomach, my head ached, I couldn't concentrate and I was scared to death. I was their elder sister and I felt I needed to be the strong one and let them know they could lean on me throughout this ordeal. I had to let them believe I was OK even though I'm not. I'm taking a page from Mom and Dad's book and I'm trying to protect Cathy and Gail. From the day each one of them came home from the hospital, like most first-born children, I assumed the role of surrogate parent. I would be responsible to watch my younger sisters when we were outside playing. When we went to school I would keep on eye on them in case they needed their big sister to intervene and I would make-up excuses (which Mom and Dad saw through anyway) to try and keep them out of trouble. I'm sure they just remember the bossiness and the tattling but I took my role as "big sister" very seriously and I worried when they were sick or late coming home from an evening out. I had a way of knowing when they were "pushing the envelope" regarding family rules and would try to give them a pre-lecture. Sometimes they listened. Sometimes they didn't; but always I was trying to be their big sister and look out for them and our family. I've always hated to see their feelings get hurt and just because we grew up doesn't make their pain any easier for me or I take my responsibility to them any less seriously. They may not need me as much now but I know I'll still want to protect them regardless of how old we get. So, what do I tell them?

Any message I send Gail she will, in turn, pass it along to Cathy since we had decided Gail would be our contact. We didn't want any of the four grandchildren to overhear our conversations until we were ready to tell them about Grandpa's health. I sat down at the computer and made several attempts to send them a message to assure them I was doing fine. I couldn't even begin to string two words together. My thoughts were so scattered.

Subject: Good Morning, Lil' Sis
Date:    2005 April 27—10:30 a.m.
From:   Susan Arnold
To:     Gail Clark

Firstly, I would like to thank you and Cathy for keeping your promise to me. I appreciate being given the facts and the time to adjust to what we may have ahead of us. Being a Girl Guide taught us to "Be Prepared". It is hard to be prepared when you are struck from behind. I'm not falling to pieces and, while I've had a few moments, I'm getting on with my day as if everything is as it should be. Naturally, Ron knows. He figured something was up from the bits and pieces he over heard but waited until I was ready to confide. We'll take one day and one step at a time. As you said last night, we are still at the investigative stage. I e-mailed Mom and Dad this morning as per usual and the tone was very light and chatty filled with tidbits from our day. I mentioned we'd like to come down for Mother's Day but to let us know if they have plans.

A quick e-mail would be great if you've heard from Mom and Dad today to let me know how they are doing (mentally and emotionally). I will call you, as we said, on Thursday evening but any little e-mail would help get me through tomorrow. The hardest part about being so far away is not being with you. Yes, that sounds like I'm stating the obvious but it is hard knowing your family is going through something scary and I'm not there to hold your hand or have mine held.

Anyway, as stated earlier, I'm doing OK. I'm your big sister and I'm here for you and Cathy. We'll deal with whatever comes down the pipe together. Thanks again for respecting our pact and making the decision to call.

Lots of love,

Susan

Gail responded with this short note:

---

Subject: Re: Good Morning, Lil' Sis
Date:    2005 April 27—13:43
From:    Gail Clark
To:      Susan Arnold

Hi, Sue;

I know that it is difficult to keep your mind from running away with all the "what ifs" and I have had some moments ... so has Cathy, but as you say, we need to put our brave faces on for Mom and Dad ... if they feel they are trying to protect you from worrying before they have the test results then let them think they have. I'll give Cathy a call today ... she's having her hair cut at 3:30 so I might see if she wants to meet for a coffee before she goes home ... she wanted to make sure you were okay. I'll talk to you soon.

Love,

Gail

Cathy did meet Gail for coffee in the afternoon and they were both relieved I was aware of what was happening. Today I have purposely not made any mention to Ron about Dad's tests or made reference to Gail's call last night. As far as I'm concerned this is a clear case of "ignore it and it will go away".

## Thursday, April 28, 2005

*Greg* and Ron are heading to Sault Ste Marie this afternoon after school. Greg and one of his hockey teammates have been invited to play in a Cancer Society three-on-three hockey tournament this weekend. How ironic! Over eighty teams are playing in all categories and Greg has been looking forward to this since the end of March.

I arrived at the South River Municipal Office, where I have been the Treasurer for the past eleven years, and found an e-mail from Gail on my computer. She had decided to sit with Mom and Cathy in the waiting room while Dad was having his procedure. Her e-mail was just filling me in on the logistics of what time Mom, Dad and Cathy were leaving Sharbot Lake for Dad's appointment at the hospital in Kingston and what time Gail was planning to be at the hospital to meet them. Basically, Gail just wanted me to have some contact with the family since she understands today will be a very long day for all of us and even more for me when I'm not with them to see what is happening. We arranged for me to call her tonight.

## 2 pm

The procedure hadn't started on time which meant Dad was prepped and waiting longer than necessary. My nerves would have been shot. I wondered how Dad was. The doctor had said not to expect to have the results today. Gail said Mom was allowed to go into the recovery room and sit with Dad until he was able to leave the hospital. Later, Dad came strolling out of the recovery area looking like he had just finished a business meeting and suggested they head to Morrison's Restaurant for lunch. His procedure meant he could only eat soft food and small amounts as he hadn't eaten since the previous evening. Instead, Gail suggested going to her house for soup and a chance to relax. Dad kept the conversation light and Gail said it was very surreal. Dad did experience some nausea and once he felt up to it Mom, Cathy and he returned home to Sharbot Lake. Our conversation was brief since Gail's head was aching badly so we hung up with promises to talk again soon.

I, actually, didn't think I would hear from Mom and Dad tonight. I thought Dad would be tired after his procedure and the travelling to Kingston for testing three days in a row not to mention all the emotions and stress associated with the tests. However, shortly after Gail and I hung up Dad and Mom called. Dad was on one phone, Mom was on an extension. Our "three ways", as we used to call them, was our usual practice when we talked on the phone. Nobody had to repeat a story twice and everyone heard the punch-line of a joke at the same time. It is a known and accepted fact in our family that Dad hates to give us bad news and always tries to soften it with normal chit-chat and all the while he is searching for just the right words to deliver what we won't want to hear. The first few minutes were passed with both of them expressing delight that we were planning a visit to Sharbot Lake on Mother's Day and discussions surrounding a leaf blower Dad had recently purchased.

Then, in his matter-of-fact way Dad told me the progression of events which lead to his tests. He told me everything, including the fact that the doctors were very certain it was malignant. I let him talk, I asked some questions but, in truth, my brain had simply gone to autopilot. Dad sounded so brave. It was like we were discussing somebody else. I don't remember a lot of the actual conversation but I do recall Dad saying something about nobody lives forever and an old tree in the forest must fall down to make way for the young saplings. That was Nature's way. I thanked them for telling me and told them we had always been a team and we would get through this together as well. We said "I love you" and ended the call.

I called Cathy to tell her that Mom and Dad had told me about Dad's lung cancer and she dissolved into tears at the sound of my voice. I tried to tell her everything would be OK but nothing seemed to stem her flow of tears. My own tears had started out of sympathy for Cathy's struggle and we finally ended the call until we were both able to speak intelligently.

My next phone call was to Gail. As soon as she heard my voice she, too, broke into tears and began apologizing. "I'm sorry, Sue, I just couldn't go against their wishes again." This reaction, on the heels of Cathy's reaction, told me something was very wrong. Obviously I had missed crucial information. I suggested she tell me *exactly* what happened at the hospital. As she retold the events of the day, everything was pretty much as Mom and Dad had said until she got to the part where the doctor had called Mom into the hospital hallway following Dad's procedure. Cathy and Gail had followed. Instead of hearing that his test was finished and Dad would be out of the recovery room shortly the doctor announced Dad had cancer of the lung and it looked fairly extensive. She felt surgery wasn't an option and our best bet would be to keep him comfortable. Mom asked if Dad had been told and the doctor indicated he was aware of their findings. Then she was gone, leaving Mom and the girls to walk back into the waiting room and absorb what they had just heard.

Mom was then allowed to go into where Dad was and they stayed there together for about twenty minutes. When Mom went into the recovery room Dad could see she had been crying and asked her what was the matter. She said the news wasn't very good. Dad didn't know what she meant and so the task fell to Mom to explain to her husband, of almost forty-nine years, what the doctor had told her. To be fair, Dad was hard of hearing and didn't have his hearing-aids in place because of the procedure and if the doctor didn't look at him directly he wouldn't have heard her. In the waiting room Cathy and Gail were trying to get a grip on their fear and but on brave faces.

Cold fear began to settle around my heart. I had enough focus to run to the bedroom to speak on the portable phone to keep Brandon, who was sitting beside me in the livingroom watching a television program, from hearing me.

"What are you saying?" The words were mine but the voice wasn't one I recognized. Gail could only cry. "What are you saying?" Again that voice asked the questions swirling in my brain. My panic caused the words to escalate in their pitch.

"Were we given any sort of a time line?"

"I don't know, Sue, maybe a year. I'm sorry I didn't tell you when we were speaking earlier. I just couldn't go against their wishes one more time."

Obviously, Dad must have thought he had told me everything but had stopped just short of telling me it was cancer. I'm not even sure how Gail and I concluded the call. I think Gail said something about going to Sharbot Lake to spend the next day with Cathy. Cathy and her husband, Steve, were going to tell the kids. Cathy and Steve couldn't hide the heartbreaking news from Lindsay and

Bradley any longer. I hung up, went back out to the livingroom and watched the rest of the program with Brandon. I felt like I was pulled in half and all that kept the two halves together was a very fine thread which could break at any moment. One half was the little girl who had just found out her Daddy was sick and the other half was the mom who needed to be brave and protect her son's feelings. When Ron called later in the evening from Sault Ste Marie he couldn't speak much since Greg was in the hotel room with him but Ron heard enough to know it was bad. I didn't tell him how bad. Time enough when they arrive home on Sunday.

### Friday, April 29, 2005

*Is* this what shock feels like? I feel like I'm watching a movie on television. I feel all the emotions and watch to see what happens next but the movie doesn't seem to end. There is no grand announcement to reveal an error, no phone call to say the test results had been read incorrectly, no happy scene with the family hugging each other while crying tears of joy. There is no reprieve.

I just don't understand why I didn't *know* something was wrong. Why didn't I *feel* something wasn't quite right? My intuition has always kicked in when talking to my family. The tone of voice, the choice of words or the slightest change in behavior had always been enough to tip me off that something wasn't as it should be. Dad and Mom had been dealing with this alone and I didn't pick up on any clues. I feel so guilty. How many things have I innocently said to them which made their secret so much more difficult to keep? Have I talked about summer plans or a special project we could do? I should have known! I just should have known!

It will be four or five business days before we hear what the tests revealed. Slowly, things are starting to register in my brain as I try to go about my day. The tests will tell us if the cancer is anywhere else in his body. We will know what, if anything, can be done for Dad. We will know how aggressive the cancer is and what kind of time frame we are looking at. Gail had said, "maybe a year." I can't remember why she said a year. Was she quoting the doctor? "Maybe a year" could also mean maybe less than a year. How much less? Six months? Two months? Everyday is a gift. Why don't we realize that more often? And why do we automatically skip over the time we have left and focus on the end? I've got to get this together. My jumbled thoughts and fears must be caged. Brandon has to go to school. He is a natural worrier and he figures things out far too quickly. I can't wake him up and have him see me in this state. He's going to his friend, Nigel's, for an overnight tonight. That means he'll have fun and not pick up clues from me. I can't tell him until Greg is home. Dad has been such a huge part of their lives. Mom and Dad were at the hospital the day each of our sons was born. We've celebrated birthdays, Christmas, Easter and Thanksgiving together. They were present for the first lost tooth with both boys. They attended hockey games and skating carnivals. Grandpa and Grandma have been with them when we've been camping, when we visited Disney Land and every other vacation we've taken. Mom and Dad took the kids on their first plane ride and witnessed their first swim in the ocean. They went for boat rides at the cottage, played at the Clark family farm in Arden and went hunting at the camp. So many activities and so many memories and so much fun together. Now we have to tell them it may all be ending far too soon. I'm not even sure how we'll find the words. I just can't think about that now.

I e-mailed Mom and Dad this morning. We've e-mailed practically every day since February 14, 2002 when Dad first went on-line, so I can't miss today or they will know why.

---

**Subject: Good Morning!**
**Date:    2005 April 29—9:12 AM**
**From:    Susan Arnold**
**To:       Harold Clark**

I hope you had a chance to get some sleep last night. I can imagine you are tired from everything leading up to our call last night and the three trips to Kingston this week.

I want to thank you for telling me and not trying to protect me by keeping this to yourselves. Everyone deals with things differently but nobody can deal with what they don't know about. I will admit my brain sort of shut down while we were talking and I don't think I've entirely processed what you said yet. I slept a bit last night and I have the office to keep my mind busy today. I will talk to you again on Sunday if not sooner.

Love to both,

Susan

---

I can't talk to anyone about this yet. I'm on the verge of tears every minute. I just know I can't handle anyone asking me about Dad. As long as I keep my mind focused on what is happening right in front of me I can push this nightmare away from my thoughts. I seem to be on some sort of emotional wave. I'm fine one second and then the next second I've dissolved into tears and the very next second I'm back to normal. I just have to focus. I just have to concentrate on every thought, every movement and every breath. If I allow myself even one unguarded moment I will simply dissolve into a puddle of tears. Much better to concentrate on moving forward through the day taking one step, one thought, one minute at a time.

I drove Brandon out to his friend Nigel's after school. He was excited and looking forward to doing some biking with Nigel. He'll be fine. I'll pick him up tomorrow around noon and we'll spend some time together in North Bay at the shopping center.

Alone at our place I made a piece of toast for dinner. I can't even begin to think about eating. I just can't swallow and when I do most things find a way of coming backup. Since Tuesday, all I've eaten are bananas, yogurt and toast. I've told both of the girls we have to take care of ourselves in order to deal with the future. Gail has Colitis and poor diet and stress exasperate the condition. In my head I know I have to get my rest, eat well and continue with my exercise routine for my own sake, for Dad and Mom's sake and for the sake of our entire family. But what my head knows my body won't allow. Perhaps this is just part of the process and once the shock has worn off I'll be able to eat again. The lump in my throat has grown to the size of an orange and there are even moments when it feels like it has become bigger than a cantaloupe. The waves of tears are continuing. As I puttered in the kitchen and tried to make the evening seem normal I picked up the wooden chopping board Dad made me as a joke gift one Christmas and the flood of emotions I had been holding back since Tuesday came rushing at me and surrounded me like a tidal wave. I sank to the floor and sat there clutching the wooden board to my breast as if it possessed the healing power to make Dad well again. Memories, thousands of them, washed through my head. The memories from a lifetime, my lifetime, tumbled over one another. The wails which came from somewhere deep inside me were almost primitive. When the storm passed I leaned against the kitchen cupboards too tired to move; too exhausted to think.

How the hell did we get here? Two months ago we were sitting in lounge chairs in Panama enjoying life without a care in the world.

## Saturday, April 30, 2005

*I* made it through today riding the same wave of emotion I've ridden for the past few days. I was able to adopt a normal demeanor and take a newspaper to my father-in-law, Allie Arnold. Brandon and I went to North Bay, Ontario Saturday afternoon and we had a really good time together. North Bay is a small city approximately seventy kilometers from South River and is home to shopping malls, movie theatres, a large selection of restaurants and several sporting facilities. Brandon told me on the way home that he enjoyed the day with me as much as he enjoyed his night at Nigel's. High praise, indeed! Brandon speaks of Grandpa and Grandma often and several times on the drive home from North Bay he mentioned them in our conversation. He would like to buy a pellet gun and he thinks he could target practice at Grandpa's farm in Arden, Ontario.

Fortunately, I was wearing sunglasses and Brandon couldn't see my face. I had completely forgotten about the farm! Dad has talked about selling his family homestead for the past several years but now I expect he'll want to do it soon. The property has so much potential and he'll want to make sure everything is tidied up and not leave the burden of selling to Mom. I may not only be losing my Dad, but the farm, too. My great-grandfather, Herbert Clark, raised his family of three boys on that farm. His son, my grandfather, lived there his entire life with two brief exceptions … nine years during the Depression when he moved to Watertown, New York and the last year before he died. My dad was raised on that property. Although my sisters and I weren't raised in Arden we were there often because Arden was only a short, twenty minute drive from Sharbot Lake. For the past twenty years we have used the farm as a recreational retreat. Our whole family gathers there for weekends in the summer and the fall. The hills are truly alive; not with the sound of music but the sound of four-wheelers and children's laughter. In any given direction my children can walk in the footsteps of four other generations. My great-grandfather's original log cabin still stands after more than a hundred years. It is a testament to the determination and the fortitude of my family's past. The connection I feel for that property is almost physical. When I feel as though life is hard I'll visit the log cabin and regain my perspective. If my great-grandparents could survive the trials which life presented them on a daily basis and raise three boys in that tiny space then I can most certainly survive what my life sets before me.

I didn't call anyone today. I couldn't trust myself to carry a conversation without breaking into tears. I need time to gather my thoughts. Ron phoned me twice today; once in the morning and once later in the evening. I'll be so glad when he is home. Ron always has a calming effect on me. I'll be better when he is with me.

## Sunday, May 1, 2005

***Brandon*** has been very good company for me and has helped without even knowing. He reminds me of Dad in so many ways. I've often remarked on the resemblance. There is something in the eyes, I think.

Gail called around noon today. She sounded tired. She said, like me, both she and Cathy have been experiencing the same emotional waves. They're fine one minute and a mess the next. Cathy's kids were told on Friday evening. They are dealing with it. As close as our boys are to Grandpa, Cathy and Steve's kids, Lindsay and Bradley, are even closer since they have always lived in Sharbot Lake, the same community as Mom and Dad. I don't think Lindsay and Bradley have ever had to deal with the frightening realities of cancer. Neither have Greg and Brandon. To our boys, cancer is not a scary, deadly disease. Grandpa Arnold had surgery to remove his bowel cancer and then he was fine. Our two boys will be told next. It is going to be difficult for all of us. Talking to Gail and Cathy helps me. We made plans for Mother's Day weekend. Cathy and Steve are going to be at Mom and Dad's when we arrive on Friday evening. I need the buffer. I'm so afraid I'll take one look at Dad and fall apart. Emotions will be running high and I want to keep it together and having Cathy and Steve there will help. I hope.

Ron and Greg arrived home from Sault Ste Marie around 2pm. Just seeing Ron come through the door was enough to bring me to tears but I recovered quickly. Greg is too tired to be told anything today and I just can't do it anyway.

When the boys disappeared to Brandon's room to play one of Brandon's new video games from our North Bay excursion Ron and I sat in the livingroom and I slowly, tearfully told him everything I had been told. When I was finished talking Ron sat in a stunned silence. There were just no words. I knew the feeling all too well. I told him we had to tell the boys since the doctor had made things sound so hopeless. We decided not to say anything on Monday evening as Greg had a tutor session at 8pm for math and that didn't really give him any time to recover from such news. Brandon had invited friends over so we didn't see the point in rushing. On Tuesday Greg had roller hockey in North Bay and Brandon wanted to go with them. We didn't feel telling them after they returned would be a good idea since it would be after nine and we'd all be tired. I think we're making excuses. If we don't tell the kids then perhaps it isn't real. We agreed we'd sit them down on Wednesday night after dinner to tell them. I asked Ron if he'd do the talking since I didn't think I'd be able to get the words out. He asked if I wanted to be there when the boys were told but I decided it would be better for them to have me express my emotions and deal with this as a family right from the start.

## Monday, May 2, 2005

*Sleep* has eluded me for another night. Just when I start to drift off to sleep the despair and emptiness begins to swell inside my head and my chest until I almost feel like I'm suffocating. Everyday other families are dealing with news like this. Yet, it feels like the whole world has changed and everyone should be as upset as I am. How dare people carry on with their normal lives while I'm barely holding my world together! I've become an actress. I put on a smile when I step out the door and make all the appropriate responses to the endless comments about the weather and pretend everything is fine. It's exhausting. I feel like a robot which has been programmed to respond positively to any and all inquiries. No emotions; just responses.

I managed to eat some mushroom soup for dinner tonight. I can't even remember if I ate anything at lunch time. I'm not hungry and the thought of food makes me nauseous. I know I have to eat but I just can't swallow. The lump in my throat is still there.

## Tuesday, May 3, 2005

*I* told our Mayor about Dad's health. The Mayor needs to know that I will be taking some personal time away from the municipal office and struggling with emotions while I am here. He was very understanding and compassionate. He told me we can make arrangements for when I need to be away.

Ron brought me a sub-sandwich for lunch today from the new bakery in the village. He has seen how little I am eating and I just know he thought he'd tempt me with something different. I ate half of it. I put the rest into the refrigerator saying I would eat it later. I never had the chance! Greg found it! I'm glad. I really don't think I could eat any more of it.

## Wednesday, May 4, 2005

---

Subject: Re; Thinking of You
Date:       2005 May 04—10:49 AM
From:      Gail Clark
To:          Susan Arnold

I know explaining this to the kids will be difficult, I'm having a hard enough time processing it inside my head much less saying it out loud. But if it helps, Dad told Cathy he actually feels better after having the test ... could be that the saline rinse helped clean his airways a bit, or, maybe he's able to relax a little now that he knows what's going on and that we know, too. There's always a chance that this is the slow moving kind and I pray that at least one piece of this nightmare will go our way. They say writing down your feelings helps you deal with emotions. You might mention that to the boys ... maybe it could help. I won't call you—but let me know tomorrow how you and they are.

I'll talk to you later,

Love,

Gail

*Gail* doesn't know yet that I have begun chronicling this family journey. I've always kept a journal and this seemed like the most natural thing for me to do. There have been days, already, when it has been the only way I have been able to make any sense out of my many, tangled thoughts. Maybe suggesting this to the boys is a good idea. Brandon loves to write. This maybe what he needs to work through his emotions when we tell them.

After dinner tonight we told the boys. It was difficult. Initially, when we called them into the livingroom, they sensed it wasn't good. They thought they were going to be lectured about something which leaves us to wonder what they've done that we haven't noticed! I had asked Ron to do the talking but somehow the words seemed to come from me. Before I started to speak I looked at their young, expectant faces and tried to remember how they looked before they were asked to accept this unbelievable truth. I told them about Grandpa's persistent cough, how his doctor wanted to see why it hadn't gone away and how the tests had revealed lung cancer. I told them Grandpa had more tests last Tuesday, Wednesday and Thursday and these tests will tell us what kind of lung cancer he has, what kind of treatments can be used, if it has gone into any other part of his body and whether it is slow or fast growing. I explained that Grandpa didn't look any different and he really wants to see us this weekend to celebrate Mother's Day. I promised that we would try to keep our life as normal as possible for as long as possible but we'll just have to take each day as it comes. We told them that it is OK to be sad but we have to try to be brave, too. As a family, ours and the extended one, we will get through this together and when one person has a bad moment the rest of us will have to be strong. Greg, at fourteen, got the seriousness of the situation immediately and sobbed while I spoke. Brandon didn't say a lot but broke into tears when he saw tears in my eyes and in his dad's. He struggled for a minute then, with twelve year-old confidence, was very adamant that Grandpa would be alright because "that's just Grandpa." He believes the doctors just have to cut the cancer out and Grandpa will be fine. We'll let this much sink in and they'll figure out the rest as we go along. Dad's doctor said the cancer in the lung was extensive and the tumor is the size of an apple. Whatever the tests reveal we're in for the fight of our lives in the next few months.

I told Ron's brother and his wife today because I don't want them hearing about it from someone else. Even though the boys aren't supposed to say anything to anyone just yet they will need their friends for support. It's only normal to confide in someone. I don't want to tell my father-in-law, Allie, before we hear the test results. He and Dad have spent many hours, over the years, visiting and discussing so many topics they found they had in common. I'd rather not say anything about Dad's diagnosis until we know everything.

Ron is just so good. He's obviously upset, just as I am, but he manages to keep the boys calm and the laundry caught up. He comforts me in so many ways and often without saying anything. The whole time he's dealing with our family crisis he still manages to work at our convenience store, The South River Kwik Way, and help out friends and family when they need him. He is one of the most thoughtful men I know and he is so strong.

*Brandon*

*One day Mom and Dad sat my brother and I down after dinner and told us Grandpa had lung cancer. Up until that point in my life I had never seen my Dad cry. That scared me. I didn't really understand how serious it was. I figured nothing bad could ever happen to Grandpa, he was never sick. If the doctor could get rid of Gampie's cancer why was it any different with Grandpa? I was up most of that night thinking of anything I could do to make everyone feel better, especially my Mom.*

## Thursday, May 5, 2005

*Today* I seem to be having a good morning, so far. I haven't dissolved into tears yet which is the first time since a week ago Tuesday. Dad left his daily e-mail this morning detailing what he and Mom are up to today. They are heading to Perth to do a bit of shopping and pick up some part for the riding lawnmower. It sounds like they are doing completely normal stuff. The trouble is nothing is normal anymore and normal things seem, somehow, abnormal in this new reality.

I came to a realization last night and it helped me make a big decision. I've decided nothing in my life has really changed yet. I'm not going to focus on the end of Dad's life and miss out on now. He could outlive all of us. Unplanned things happen. If Dad is given two years to live or one year or less I'm not going to mourn him before he is gone and lose this opportunity to build memories with all my family; my husband, my boys, both my parents, my sisters and their families. We'll have tough times ahead but for now we're all still here. I'm not going to fear the future because that is what it is … the future. Right now I'm working on autopilot. Thinking of a future without Dad in it brings me to the edge of tears but for the moment we're still whole. We're also extremely fortunate. Dad mentioned that this could have happened when he and Mom had a young family but he's been blessed with time to enjoy life and develop relationships with not only his wife and children but with his grandchildren. He is so wise and he's being so unbelievably strong. Is it real? Is he in denial? How can we really be sure what thoughts are privately held? Regardless, Dad has a valid point about our family's good fortune. We have been blessed. We've never had to deal with anything as serious as Dad's illness. We lost people we loved but our family unit seemed to have been blessed with good health and time. The time we have doesn't have to be spent mending fences. We've always said "I love you." We've always said "I'm proud of you." We don't get together just for the special occasions because "we should" we invent special occasions so "we can" get together. We've collected good memories. We were taught to take some risks in life and to dream and work to make the dream come true. We were also taught to appreciate what we have; not what we would like to have. We learned life is only worth living with family and true friends to share it. We have what many will never have. Dad has always told us "things happen for a reason." I've relied on his good sense too many times in my life to start forgetting what he has taught me now.

I have to pack for the weekend. We're planning to leave for Sharbot Lake by 3:30 p.m. or 4:00 p.m. tomorrow. Cathy and Gail want me to bring brie, garlic and crackers to have with drinks before dinner. Dad, especially, liked the roasted garlic and brie cheese when I've served it in the past. Cathy is cooking a turkey and Gail is making some salads. I'll help with the meal preparation and the clean up.

I had a massage this afternoon which has helped relax me. My back muscles were one huge knot and the massage got rid of the pain.

I am impatient and want to be at Mom and Dad's in Sharbot Lake, now!

## Friday, May 6, 2005

**Subject: Morning**
**Date:    2005 May 06—08:31**

From:    Gail Clark
To:        Susan Arnold

Hi, Sue;

Thanks for the call last night—didn't mean to sound "down" but I'd had a long day and what you heard in my voice was tired as much as anything. Anyway, the reason for this morning's message is to tell you I called Mom and Dad last night. When they returned from Cathy's there was a message on their machine from the Specialist's office. They have an appointment set for Dad at 2:45 p.m. today to discuss his test results.

Dad isn't too impressed at the prospect of heading back to Kingston again today and his first inclination was to call and say he wasn't coming until next week ... but the message also said something about the doctor being away for a while.

I'm sure that the appointment is weighing on his mind so he might better hear what she has to say instead of waiting. I asked them to call Cathy and ask her to come into the appointment with them and help decipher what they're told—of course they didn't want to interrupt her day but I think they did decide to call her last night. I'll find out the plan and when I know I'll e-mail you. I'd like to go, too, just to hear for myself what's being said so I don't get a watered down version. Mom said she expects they will be home long before you get there but if, for any reason, they are delayed you have a key.

Anyway, I'll call Cathy now and then I'll get back to you.

I'll be in touch.

Love,

Gail

***Concentrating*** at work today was especially difficult. Part of the problem was in knowing I would actually be in Sharbot Lake before the end of the day. I've wanted to be there since last Tuesday and now I'm just unbelievably antsy. The other part of the problem was getting the news via Gail's e-mail saying the doctor wanted to see Dad and Mom this afternoon. Both Cathy and Gail were able to arrange to go into the appointment with Mom and Dad. Apparently Dad told one doctor "the Clark family travels in a pack so I'll always have one or more of my family with me at these appointments."

Travelling to Sharbot Lake was very difficult for Ron, the boys and I. We knew the family already knew Dad's prognosis. What if we find out when we arrive home that Dad has only a short time? What if the cancer has spread to other parts of his body? What would we find? So many thoughts and memories crowded into my brain as we travelled the many miles toward my hometown. I hid behind my sunglasses as I had so many other times this past week. I hide so people can't see the haunted look of fear in my eyes or the red rims from crying. I hide so I can pretend I don't see someone which would result in some conversation. And, I am afraid to go home. I am afraid of the news. I am afraid of how I'll react. I've never been afraid of going home. Home has always been a sanctuary, a welcoming place of love and security. Already this disease has robbed me of that one constant in my life. What else will it take from us before we're through? By the time we stopped in Bancroft for gas I couldn't stand it anymore. I had to know what was going on. I just couldn't walk into that house not knowing what the doctor had said. I took the cell phone and went to the furthest part of the parking lot and called Cathy.

Cathy almost seemed like she was waiting for my call and answered on the first ring. She told me they all felt much better when they left the doctor's office and that she'd let Dad and Mom tell me everything.

"No! You have to tell me. Is there a time frame? Is it in other parts of his body? This trip has been unbearable. I can't travel another mile without hearing what happened at the doctor's office!"

Cathy was great. She told me there isn't a time frame. Dad has Non-Small Cell Cancer on a third of his superior lobe on his left lung. His cancer is slow growing and there didn't appear to be evidence that it had spread into his liver, spleen or adrenal glands but further testing was required to be conclusive. His breathing capacity is good although his left lung is partially collapsed. Cathy also said there was even a slight possibility of radiation and/or surgery which could result in a cure. Cure? Surely the doctor hadn't used the word cure? How is that possible when the first doctor told Dad to put his affairs in order if he hadn't already taken those planning measures. Certainly this was more hope than the doctor had first given us. Both Cathy and Gail took notes so I could read everything the doctor had said and Dad and Mom could reread the notes in case they had missed something or forgot the answer. Clever thinking on both their parts and something we have decided to do with each future visit.

The doctor had scheduled the bone scan with radioactive material and a complete body scan for Monday morning. By the time Cathy finished telling me that Mom and Dad were doing OK, and were cautiously optimistic, I was trembling so badly I could barely standup. I hurried back to the truck to tell Ron and the boys what Cathy had said.

The rest of the trip to Sharbot Lake took on a more normal atmosphere. We played our usual travelling games and I felt as if we could plan events this summer with Dad participating. He could attend Gail's graduation in June and perhaps spend a weekend at our cottage. Above all, we had hope and, apparently, we had time.

Walking into the house on this first visit since hearing of Dad's illness was highly charged and full of emotion but we tried, for all our sakes, to keep things fairly low key. We each knew that if one person broke down we all would and I could see Mom and Dad were very tired. Both Mom and Dad welcomed me home with a hug which almost seemed as though they were giving me some of their strength. Cathy and Steve and the kids were there which really helped get our visit on track quickly. As we chatted about our trip it was hard to believe Dad had any sort of an illness. I sat next to Dad's chair and watched him closely while he spoke. I looked at every inch of his face and his neck searching for something which suggested Dad's health was compromised. What had I missed seeing? Surely something as serious as lung cancer would have given us some visual clues. Everything about Dad suggested a healthy man was sitting next to me. I was almost able to lull myself into the belief that Dad wasn't as ill as I had been told. Surely everyone had simply overreacted. Then, he coughed and the room became silent. It was the same hollow-sounding cough we had heard since before Christmas. At Christmas it was "just a cough"; an irritant. Now, it had taken on a life of its own; it was sinister and menacing. Now, the cough became the symbol of our enemy.

While I was watching Dad I was also watching our sons, Greg and Brandon, and their reactions. I wanted to make sure they were OK. Brandon was very quiet. He sat away from the rest of us and watched everything that was going on. He was doing the same thing I had done; he was sizing up the situation. The Grandpa he always knew was sitting before him and he was trying to understand how this man could be the Grandpa we had told him about earlier this week. Greg sat with Grandma and Aunt Cathy and told them and Grandpa all about his recent trip to Sault Ste Marie. Then the boys disappeared with their cousins, Lindsay and Bradley, to talk amongst themselves.

Cathy and Steve didn't stay long after we arrived. They knew we wanted to have sometime with Mom and Dad and everyone was tired so before long we all decided to turn in early and get up in the morning rested and ready to visit. Both Dad and Mom were looking forward to our family gathering tomorrow and the turkey dinner at the end of the day. Ron and I had come up to bed feeling more relaxed then we had in a while. It helped to see both Mom and Dad but the news from the doctor's appointment had helped, too. We had options. Dad talks openly about his cancer but doesn't dwell on it. He seems to have come to terms with the illness. He's also ready to fight this monster. His head seems to be in a good place.

## Saturday, May 7, 2005

*I* heard both Mom and Dad off and on all through the night. I wasn't awake but, apparently, I wasn't completely asleep either. I remember thinking they must be having trouble sleeping.

Next morning I went downstairs ahead of the rest of my family. I wanted to have Mom and Dad all to myself. Just as I came into the kitchen I was aware of several things at the same moment. Mom's very strained look, my niece, Lindsay, and her friends arriving at the kitchen door and Dad lying on the couch in the family room talking to Cathy on the phone. There was no guess work required. He was in pain.

Dad had been up all night with a severe pain in his right side. Could it be appendices? He didn't seem to be fevered nor was he nauseous but I wasn't a nurse. Cathy was and she suggested taking him to the Medical Center in Sharbot Lake to see his doctor when it opened at 10am. In the mean time she prescribed a cold ice pack. No heat!

At 9:45am we took Dad to the Medical Center to be there when the doctor arrived. I know everyone had a small thought lurking somewhere in their consciousness that Dad's pain was somehow related to the cancer. We were sure it wasn't but there was just the smallest part of us which thought, *maybe*. Dad was the first patient Dr Bell saw and Mom went into the office with Dad. Ron and I wandered around outside waiting for word then went back inside to sit down out of the blackflies. Gail was due to leave Kingston for Sharbot Lake around noon and I suddenly thought she shouldn't leave until she knew if we were heading into Kingston to the hospital. I went outside to the car to call Cathy to find out if she'd been in touch with Gail. Gail had called for another reason and Cathy brought her up to-date on what had taken place and told her to sit tight. Cathy would tell her more when she knew more. Just as we were on the phone Mom, Dad and Ron came out of the doctor's office. I asked them if we were heading to Kingston and they said no. I told Cathy I'd call as soon as we got back to Mom and Dad's. The doctor had done several tests and determined it was a kidney stone. Of all the damn luck! One of his scans last week had shown stones in some tube. Now, one of the stones was on the move. The doctor gave Dad a shot of Demerol and suggested waiting it out at home. Dr Bell sent his personal phone number home with Dad and also promised to check in from time to time to see how Dad was and if further medical attention was needed.

Dad was weak, racked with pain and the Demerol made his stomach upset. He looked so pale and helpless as he lay on his bed. He felt so bad this had to happen on the weekend when everyone was home. Cathy and I assured him this wasn't anything which could be planned and everyone understood. It was just very bad timing. Dad was disappointed because he wanted the weekend to be somewhat normal and to allow us time, as a family, to adjust to his illness. Dad's thoughts have always been for us and our feelings, "our" being Mom, Susan, Cathy and Gail. Now "our" has been expanded to include my husband Ron, our two boys, Greg and Brandon, Cathy's husband, Steve, their children, Lindsay and Bradley and Gail's partner, Rob. He fought the Demerol for a while but eventually fell into sleep. His knees were no longer drawn up in pain and he seemed to be more comfortable.

During the day we took turns checking in on him. When he was awake we'd sit with him on the bed just like we used to do when we were little girls. Our whole family would gather onto Mom and Dad's bed after church on Sunday, once we'd changed into our play clothes, and we would make plans for the day or just talk. The grandchildren drifted in and out of his room. They didn't want to disturb Grandpa but they needed to make sure he was OK. His bedroom became the centre of the house and we joked with him about being so pampered.

Dad didn't feel up to coming downstairs for our turkey dinner. Steve carved the turkey and the rest of us tried to pretend we were having a good time but Dad's misery upstairs simply underscored his illness even though one had nothing to do with the other. Dad just wasn't there with us and yet we were all thinking about him. It was horrible. I couldn't eat a bite of the wonderful meal so I sat at the kid's table. They wouldn't notice what I did or didn't eat.

## Sunday, May 8, 2005

***Everyone*** started out the morning by visiting Dad while he was still in bed. I know having us around him makes him so happy but he really doesn't like being fussed over and, besides, it was Mother's Day; Dad felt Mom should be the one who is fussed over.

When Mom and I went into the kitchen, Gail had already made the coffee which we could smell before we got to the hallway. She had also poured a bowl of cereal and sliced a banana on top and told Mom she'd made breakfast! It was a really nice gesture which made us laugh.

Cathy arrived while we finished our toast and we all sat at the kitchen table drinking our coffee and chatting. This is a normal morning ritual when we all get together. How can we possibly find so much to say to each other after so many years? We just never seem to run out of topics.

Dad found his way downstairs and gave Mom her Mother's Day gift. I don't think he has missed an occasion in all the years of their marriage. He is such a romantic. We've been on holidays with Mom and Dad in some far away place when Valentine's Day has rolled around. Dad and Mom will have brought their cards from home and exchanged them before breakfast. They never forget an occasion. Dad bought Mom a lovely gold rope chain which she immediately put on. The rest of us each took our turn presenting Mom with her gifts and cards. It was wonderful. Dad looked somewhat better but still hadn't passed the evil kidney stone. It had probably moved into his bladder so the pain wasn't as intense. This was likely the calm before the storm.

Time was ticking away and Ron and I both knew we had to start thinking about getting packed up and leaving for South River. The road to South River is a long one although it has never seemed as long as it does now. Steve, Brad and Lindsay all arrived and we moved the gathering into the familyroom. Dad had disappeared upstairs only to return dressed for the day. He was still pale and tired-looking, but much more comfortable. It was time for us to head home. We really hated to leave when Dad wasn't feeling great but Gail was going to spend the day with them and Cathy would pop in from time to time to check on him. It's nice to have a registered nurse in the family.

Our trip home was pleasant. Gail's Rob had prepared a CD of pictures from our Panama trip and I viewed the slideshow as we travelled the many kilometers to South River. Rob did a great job in capturing the family, the resort, the scenery and life in Panama. The smiling, relaxed faces of our family looking out at me from each of the pictures had no way of knowing the tears and heartbreak that was waiting for them only a few months away.

Ron suggested an early supper when we were just outside of Bancroft. We stopped at MacDonald's. We hadn't stopped there in a long time and it really was nice to be with my guys.

We arrived home around 6:30pm and I called back to Sharbot Lake to let them know we were off the roads. This is a family rule. We always call when we arrive at our destination. I especially didn't want Mom and Dad to worry about anything more then they already had on their plate. Sometimes I unpack and make a coffee before calling but tonight I wanted them to know we were off the road as soon as possible. Mom answered and Gail picked up on the extension. Dad was resting comfortably but Mom sounded stressed. More than when we had left. I was so tired and after hanging up the phone I fell asleep on the couch. I was just bone weary and couldn't hold my eyes open. My head had started to ache someplace along the road. The events leading up to the weekend and the weekend itself with the optimistic news on Friday combined with Dad's kidney stone misery was emotionally exhausting. How will I ever get through what lies ahead for our family when I don't seem to be made of the strength I always thought I had in reserve. Perhaps I'm just being too hard on myself. Shock and emotions are very tiring. Maybe I just need to give myself permission to experience everything I'm feeling. Maybe I'll draw strength from deep within but first I have to get all of these other feelings out of the way.

*Brandon*

*The first time we went to visit Grandpa and Grandma after we knew about the cancer he seemed normal, like nothing had changed. Except, when we got there; he hugged me tighter then usual.*

*After seeing him, and knowing he was alright, I felt a lot better. The next morning was a whole different story! Grandpa was in a whole lot of pain. He was all curled up on the couch in the living room and was as white as a ghost. Nobody knew what was wrong. Finally Grandpa's doctor told him it was a kidney stone and gave him medicine to take away the pain. Grandpa slept most of the weekend and when he was awake we'd sneak in for a visit. He felt so bad about being sick while the family was there. We made plans for all of our family to go to the farm in Arden for the weekend in a couple of weeks.*

## Monday, May 9, 2005

*My* head was aching so badly I thought someone was using a jack hammer at my temples. I drove the boys to the bus and called the municipal office to say I wouldn't be in today. I just needed to sleep and get rid of this horrible tension headache.

I knew Gail would be at home today and around noon I called her to see if she heard how Dad had spent the night. Did he pass that damned stone? Also, he was scheduled for two more tests today. He will have a complete body scan to determine if the cancer was in any other organ of the body and a bone scan with radioactive material to ascertain if the cancer was in his bones. There was even some question as to whether the tests would be done if he was still in a lot of pain because of the stone. However, the tests did proceed and he had a three hour wait between being injected with the radioactive material and the time when the bone scan could be done so they drove over to Gail's.

Gail said Mom and Dad had just left her place to go back to the hospital. Apparently everything was on schedule and the scan had even been early. Sitting for endless hours in a waiting-room can be so exhausting. The stone was still inside Dad but the pain had subsided although he was still taking Demerol. The organ scan would also show the appendix. Doctor Bell had requested they look at the appendix to make sure it wasn't appendicitis. Gail said Dad had a little rest on her couch while she, Mom and Cathy chatted in the livingroom.

Gail told me Mom had a bad time yesterday afternoon. Dad's pain had come back and he had been really suffering again. Seeing him like that set off a whole train of thoughts which she shared with Gail. None of the thoughts were very optimistic but all were things she needed to deal with. She really hasn't had a lot of time on her own because she has been with Dad and he's been so strong. He only seems to get upset when he sees Mom or one of us get upset. So, she has tried to hide how scared she really is. I think the chat with Gail was good for her but it certainly explained why she sounded so strained on the phone. That, and when I called, she was with Dad in their room.

By this evening I was starting to feel better. Ron put a frozen pizza in the oven for the boys and we just ate some toast or crackers. Neither one of us was very hungry. I didn't go to Council tonight. As the municipality's Treasurer I don't miss very many meetings so I think I'm entitled. I couldn't have sat through the meeting anyway. While the headache wasn't as bad as it had been, it was still pounding across my forehead. An early night will be the best medicine.

### Tuesday, May 10, 2005

---

Subject: Good Morning
Date:   Tuesday, May 10, 2005 11:33 a.m.
From:   Susan Arnold
To:     Gail Clark

Hi, Lil' Sis;

When you're talking to Cathy next time (in case it is before I am) would you please tell her I forgot to give her the money for the theatre tickets and I'll give it to her the next time I'm down.

Mom and Dad called last night. They sounded tired but glad their day in Kingston was over.

I have a confession to make to you. I took yesterday off and wasn't just on my lunch break when I called your place. I didn't say anything because I didn't want Mom and Dad to start worrying about me. My head was aching so badly I knew there wasn't any point in going to work. I just needed to rest. Something I haven't done much of since this nightmare started. Much like everyone else in the family has experienced.

Ron and I talked last night and I told him I had figured out part of why I'm feeling it so necessary to be physically with Mom, Dad, Cathy and you. It isn't because I feel out of the loop because you and Cathy have been great. It is just a need I have to be near all of you because that is how it has always been. It doesn't matter if we talk or spend it in the waiting room I just need to be close by. I know it sounds selfish but it is more for me then for anyone else. When Ron's dad was diagnosed with cancer Ron could leave the store whenever he felt he needed to spend time with Allie and he could sit with his dad for ten or fifteen minutes and then return to work. And, he could do that as often as he wanted to. I can't. Calling on the phone doesn't seem to help because I don't really have anything to say. Ron told me to figure out what I need to do and we'll make it happen.

Obviously, since we received the good news that Dad's cancer is the slow growing kind I won't take long periods of time off of work right away but I've been toying with the idea of asking council for a couple of days a month to be used when I feel the need. I know they'll agree but I want to get written permission. Once I know what I'm doing I'll let you know. I'd be down on the weekend except I have a doctor's appointment on Monday in Toronto.

Here's a little chuckle to brighten your day. Our dog Casper returned from the kennel a different pup. I had asked them to shampoo and clip him (I forgot to add clip his toenails). Well, he looks like a freakishly large cat without fur! Not even his tail was spared! The boys couldn't believe their eyes. On the up side ... the black-flies won't burrow into his hair and he'll be cooler!

I hope you're having a good day. E-mail or call whenever you want/can. I know you know this but, for the record, I love you.

Susan

Gail understood my need to be with Mom and Dad.

---

Subject: Re: Good Morning
Date:    2005 May 10—13:43
From:    Gail Clark
To:      Susan Arnold

Hi, Sue;

I was just speaking to Cathy ... she said she just hung up from talking to you. I don't have any news but wanted to touch base.

I know what you mean about feeling like you need to do something when there's really nothing that can be done. Pray we get the referral to Dr. Reid ... he may pull the rug from under us with his opinion but at least it will mean that all the news which reached him was positive and hopeful.

I hope Mom and Dad will be able to go to the Grand Theatre on Sunday evening ... if that damn kidney stone is stubborn I don't know how long they'll leave him suffering with it before they do something. There other options from what I've read and none sound too nice (involving catheter, etc) but at least it would be over.

**I think your plan to approach council is good.**

**Take care of yourself and for the record ... I love you, too!**

**Gail**


I spoke to Cathy at length today. We discussed the tests Dad had yesterday. He will be referred to the surgeon only if the bone scan comes back clear and there isn't any other sign of cancer in his body. We have no idea how long until we hear the results but we suspect it will be by the end of the week or early next week. Everything has been fast tracked so far.

My sisters, Mom and I had selected the last weekend of May to meet for our annual Mother/Daughter Weekend in Oshawa, Ontario. We all look forward to this girls-weekend away every year. If things are good we may go ahead with the weekend. Ron and the boys said they'd go to Sharbot Lake and all the men of the family could do something together.

Here at home I made the decision to get back into the swing of things. My boys need their mother to function like a real person. I also realize how very precious every minute is to a family and I want to be sure our kids have good memories of their childhood despite this difficult time. We've tried to be good parents and have done many things with the kids to make their childhood special but it's the little things I recall from my own childhood which really stands-out in my memory. Things like homemade cookies, good night kisses and supper on the table. So, I came home prepared to get back to normal. I made poached chicken, rice and vegetables for dinner. After, I cleaned the refrigerator from top to bottom, cleaned the corner cupboard, made chicken salad for Brandon's lunch, did the dishes, made muffins and vacuumed the livingroom rug. By the time Ron and Greg came back from roller hockey in North Bay the kitchen and the livingroom were spotless. Brandon had a friend come to our house to play video games and all of us seemed to be back into a more relaxed frame of mind.

I just realized I haven't cried once today. Life is what it is. Bad things happen but there is always hope. Whatever happens; we'll be OK.

## Wednesday, May 11, 2005

*Dad* passed his kidney stone around 4am this morning. Thank God.

## Thursday, May 12, 2005

*I* missed writing an entire entry yesterday because I was busy and didn't have anything to say. The shock has worn off, I think, and the waves of emotion seem to have subsided and life seems more or less normal. Dad's cancer is never far from my mind but we seem to be learning how to live with it. In a way, it doesn't feel real. It's hard to think of Dad as being seriously ill. When I least expect it the reality of Dad's illness hits me and I continue to ask, "How the Hell did we get here?"

After dinner Ron, Casper and I took a drive to the cottage. Our cottage is located on Eagle Lake, a short drive from our home. From the end of June until Labour Day Weekend we live at the cottage and commute to work from there. I look forward to our time at the cottage long before the snow melts. I took some of the treasures I had brought back from our winter trip to Panama. I'm trying to give the cottage a tropical feel. We have had such good times in the tropics. I met Ron in the Bahamas and our large extended family has made several trips to the Caribbean together so it seems only fitting that we associate good times with both the cottage and the tropics. The cottage's current color scheme is marine-blue and red but I've decided I can add a few hits of yellow, green and orange to really liven it up. I'll add some wicker, put the oil painting I brought back from Dominican Republic on the wall and we'll display our shell collection. I don't know how much time I/we will have at the cottage this summer but while we're there it will be a happy, fun place to restore our spirits.

When we returned home from the cottage Ron took Casper for a walk and I started to clean the kitchen and baked some blueberry muffins. Greg had to go to his tutor for an hour. Ron went to visit with his dad who lives in the same community as we live. Actually, both of Ron's brothers made their homes in South River so the Arnold family is all nearby. We've decided we need to tell Allie about Dad's cancer since several people know and we don't want him to hear it from someone else. I talked to Gail at length tonight. She seemed to feel the need to retrace every event and conversation, every emotion and thought since we found out about this nightmare. I'm glad she can get it out. I know her boyfriend, Rob, is there for her but sometimes you can only express yourself to someone who has known you all your life. We laughed, we were serious and we were very grateful when she told me Dad had e-mailed her to say he had gotten the referral to Dr Reid who is the surgeon. That would indicate, to us, that Dad's bones and other organs are cancer free. His appointment is scheduled for Wednesday, May 18th at 9:30am. I hope what he has to say is promising.

Just after I hung up from Gail, Dad and Mom called to tell me about his pending appointment. Dad sounded positive but he won't let himself, or us, get our hopes built up too high. He's adopted a "wait and see" attitude. As they talked about the appointment I looked up to find Ron, Greg and Brandon gathered around the kitchen table waiting to hear what was being said. The concern was written all over their faces.

I think we'll all sleep a little better tonight.

### Friday, May 13, 2005

*I* can't believe it's been a week since we were preparing to leave for Sharbot Lake. That was a horrible trip which ended with a small amount of hope being given to our family.

I have my annual appointment at the Women's College Hospital in Toronto, Ontario on Monday morning. I'm travelling to Toronto with Ron's sister-in-law, Dawn, and her daughter, Melody, on Sunday. Last month we had booked some treatments at the Elmwood Spa for Sunday afternoon. I'm scheduled for a Moor Mud Body Wrap. I've never been wrapped in mud before but the child in me is looking forward to the experience! We're staying at our favorite spot, The Cambridge Suites, in downtown Toronto. The hotel is close to the theater, great restaurants, the spa and the hospital. Cara, Dawn's other daughter, will meet us there. I'm proud of the relationship I have with my Arnold family. I enjoy spending time with Ron's nieces, Cara and Mel. They are interesting, lovely young women and I have come to regard them as my own nieces, too. Their mother, Dawn, and I have much in common and I'm looking forward to our time away. Maybe I'll be able to think about something other than Dad's lung cancer.

Writing this journal seems to have helped me come to terms with what is going on in our lives. When I reread the earlier entries I see how far I have come in accepting Dad's illness. Given the fact it has only been two weeks I think perhaps I'm not doing too badly after all. The lump in my throat seems to have disappeared. My appetite has gotten better but still isn't back to normal. But, as long as I eat good things my diminished appetite might be a good thing! I'm sleeping better and I've gotten control of my emotions. I'm not quite so teary-eyed. We have been a very blessed family my entire life. I guess I'm getting ready for the next round; whatever that might be. Dr Reid's appointment is crucial to finding out what can be done for Dad, and when. If Dad undergoes radiation or chemo-therapy, we'll have to brace ourselves for the side effects which accompany those processes. We just have to remember to take things one step and one day at a time.

## Tuesday, May 17, 2005

*I* had a really nice weekend. It was very eventful and productive. On Saturday afternoon, after Ron and the boys returned from roller hockey, Ron and I decided to do some yard-work at the cottage. We raked over half the yard and bagged the leaves as we went. I really feel good about getting so much done.

Back at home, Ron took Casper for a walk and I sorted my winter clothes, packed a box for charity and put my summer clothes into the drawers. I also packed my suitcase for Toronto so I felt like I had done a lot.

Mel picked me up Sunday morning around 8:30am. Dawn was ready when we arrived at their place. The drive to Toronto went quickly. We arrived at the hotel around noon and were able to get into our room. We freshened up from our travels and then walked the few blocks to the Elmwood Spa.

I have never had a body wrap and the experience was quite interest-ing. First, most of my body was painted with black, clay-like mud from the Dead Sea. Then, I was wrapped in a large sheet of plastic to induce sweating. The sweating would release toxins from the skin. On top of me were piled four or five layers of blankets to increase the temperature inside my muddy cocoon. My head was covered with a towel and moistened gauze was placed over my eyes. Then the lights were dimmed and I was to be left alone for about twenty-minutes to sweat, rest and relax.

Apparently I have claustrophobia!

I felt trapped and desperate! In a shrill, high-pitched voice, that didn't sound quite so shrill or high-pitched in my mind, I politely screamed that I didn't think I could be left by myself for such a long time! The esthetician very quickly removed the cloth from my eyes, massaged my head and told me to take several long, deep breathes. "Take a deep breath, now relax and let it out. Take a deep breath, now relax and let it out. And again." Eventually, I did feel better and was able to tolerate the rest of the session. Note to myself: *No more body wraps!*

After leaving the spa we went shopping for a couple of hours. Nothing seemed to call out to me! Perhaps I'm still in shock because I always have an interest in shopping! I did manage to find a present and a card for Gail's university graduation. Funny, I found choosing the card more difficult then I imagined. The experience was similar to buying a Mother's Day card for Mom. Our family always chooses cards which seem to be written by us with sentiments which come from our hearts. All of the graduation cards were talking about bright futures, dreams, having it all, etc. They just didn't seem right given the current situation. Card companies should introduce a selection of cards that express sentiments for those times when life isn't all roses and rainbows. Eventually, I did manage to find one which said how proud we were of her and how special she is to us. My dilemma was solved.

We had dinner reservations at Baton Rouge and I ordered a drink and a spinach salad with a salmon fillet. The salad was very good but far too big for me to finish. Following dinner the girls and I went to a corner store and bought some snacks to eat while we watched the movie, *Spanglish*, with Adam Sandler. By the time it was over I was ready for bed. The next morning would be an early start.

Our breakfast arrived around the same time our wake up call came through. We were organized and managed to get everyone showered, dressed and packed before we took our cab to the hospital for our appointments. Things moved quickly and there wasn't a lot of wait-time which was nice.

We had made arrangements to meet back at the hotel lobby. While waiting in the lobby for the girls to return Dawn and I saw Kate Hudson, her husband, baby and entourage. They were in the lobby getting checked in. She is much smaller in person and very young looking. The Cambridge Suites is a hotel which is quiet, dignified and elegant. It is located in the heart of downtown Toronto but a bit off the beaten track so their privacy would be assured.

We said good-bye to Cara and began the three hour return trip home to South River. I was very tired and had developed a headache but I did enjoy myself much more than I had thought I would. I'm glad I didn't cancel my appointment as I had decided I would shortly after hearing Dad's news. I had a few moments over the weekend when Dad's illness weighed heavily on my heart but I was able to bring myself under control very quickly.

When I'm away I really miss my guys and I was happy to hear all about their activities while I was away from them. With everything going on I realize just how much I love my husband and our boys and, despite their own sadness, they are giving me great strength.

---

**Subject: Re: Good morning!**
**Date:** 2005 May 17—10:47
**From:** Harold Clark
**To:** Susan Arnold

Hi, Susan!

Glad to hear that you are home safe and sound from Toronto and that you've had good medical reports and a good time. As for the mud treatment; we can recall seeing you in similar circumstances years ago but never in a thousand years could we picture you now in that cloak!!! Oh, well—if it turns your crank!

We are really glad to hear of Greg's math marks and in passing his assignments. Tell him we feel he did this for us and we know he will continue. He just needs to have his confidence built up, as we know he can do it.

Mom is busy doing her routine things and I'm still the supervisor. We are getting along fine and will be in touch tomorrow evening after we get back from Kingston.

So, for now, take care. Have a good day and say hi to all.

Love Mom and Dad

### Wednesday, May 18, 2005

*I'm* finding the waiting difficult today. Dad's appointment with Dr Reid, the surgeon, was scheduled for 9:30am this morning. I've been watching the clock every minute as well as the computer for some word on how the meeting went. I know Dad said he'd call me tonight but I just can't wait that long. Gail wasn't going to the meeting this time but Cathy was. She will be their stenographer. Cathy will write down what the doctor says so Mom and Dad have a written record of the conversation to study after they leave the appointment. Also, as Dad said to Gail, having Cathy there keeps him "honest." In other words, he can't give us a watered down version of what was said to keep us from worrying too much. At this point, I don't think he'd do that. He wants Mom to have as much support as possible and keeping us in the dark about his cancer would prevent our full support. I keep thinking I should be praying every minute of the day. Praying God will spare my father's life. Our faith has always been very deep and quiet and right now I don't feel the need to pray because I know God will do what is right. I have asked Him for strength and to help Dad and our family travel this journey together.

It's now 12:30pm. The appointment was three hours ago. What was said? What was decided? It was my Dad's health being discussed but it was our family's life which will be effected by the decisions. I have nothing more to write but somehow the act of writing and thinking about them makes me feel closer to them.

## Thursday, May 19, 2005

*Dad's* appointment didn't give us the result we had expected and, in fact, underscored the severity of his disease. Dr Reid does not recommend surgery. The surgery is very risky and Dad might not make it through the operation to remove one entire lung. The risks post-operative are many and not infrequent. On top of all that, he would need to recover from the surgery and then undergo chemotherapy and radiation in an already weakened condition. The outcome of the surgery isn't a guarantee either. Dad would likely be a respiratory invalid, incapable of moving, laughing and talking. Dad wouldn't live long like that. He'd go raving mad. So, the option, for the time being, is a combination of radiation and chemotherapy probably starting in the next couple of weeks. We really don't have a lot of time. Years go by quickly and, at best, we probably only have a couple of years together.

Gail and I talked for almost two hours after Dad and Mom called us. We are disappointed but, perhaps, this is the better way after all. I've decided I'm not past the shock of all this. I'm numb. The tears have stopped, for the most part, and now all I'm left with is a time-less state where only this moment exists. I feel like I'm hanging on a string and I'm being blown in several directions with no time to react.

My sisters and I have to make sure Dad's quality of life is the best it can possibly be. We want to continue to do the things which make Dad and Mom happy and continue to fill our family-memory bank with wonderful times. Heaven knows there will be enough bad times ahead. Chemotherapy is no picnic.

I spoke to Cathy in the afternoon and Mom and Dad right after dinner. Gail called in the evening so we were all in contact today. This morning, when I went to the store to get my coffee, Ron suggested I go to Sharbot Lake for the long weekend. At first, I thought it was a good possibility. Now, I'm not sure. I don't want Mom and Dad to think they are living in a fishbowl and need to be babysat. Also, they would feel uncomfortable if they thought we were changing our lives too much when nothing has really changed. Nothing, that is, except our entire world.

I feel so helpless. I can't even make them a casserole. Talking on the phone is fairly stilted. Dad tries to make the cancer the smallest part of our conversations but it is very much the elephant-in-the-room. Talking about Greg's success on his recent math test and Brandon's grade six testing seems so strange. I suppose Dad needs to pretend things are normal.

## May 19, 2005

---

Village of South River
Personnel Committee
C/O J. Coleman

Dear Jim;

I'm writing to advise you that my father was diagnosed at the end of April with lung cancer. Surgery is not an option and he will be starting chemotherapy shortly. I expect to be spending many weekends in the foreseeable future at my parents' in Sharbot Lake. There may be times when my family needs me to be with them during the week. I am requesting permission, in advance, to use my vacation time and to take unpaid personal time when necessary and upon short notice.

Our family's goal is to keep life as normal as possible for as long as possible therefore the necessity of taking weekdays off at present should be minimal. Every effort will be made not to have the Village's routine disrupted for personal reasons.

I hope that you and the rest of Council will find these arrangements satisfactory and I thank you in advance for your support during this time.

Sincerely,

Susan

## Friday, May 20, 2005

---

Subject: Re: Good Morning
Date:    2005 May 19—12:21
From:   Harold Clark
To:      Susan Arnold

Hi, Susan!

We are experiencing the same kind of weather as you are but it's suppose to improve as the week goes on. We aren't over run with black flies, as yet, however our turn is coming.

Mom and I have been out in the yard seeding where it showed signs of winter kill. Mom took a bunch of dandelions out with the picker that we got in town yesterday. I used it after we got home. It works but it doesn't make the job any easier.

We may take a drive down to Perth this afternoon ... pick up a few things and see the folks. Nothing else here so we'll run along.

Take care and we will be talking to you later.

Love Mom and Dad

---

The word is out.

Mom and Dad went to Perth, Ontario, a small town located forty kilometers east of Sharbot Lake to see one of Mom's sisters and to tell her about Dad's cancer. Then, they stopped at Uncle Art and Aunt Sue's. Uncle Art is Mom's older brother and the two couples have been good friends over the years.

Since Uncle Art's retirement they have spent many hours with Mom and Dad. The four of them have travelled from Newfoundland, Canada to Texas, United States. They've been all over the Caribbean together and have visited our cottage in 2004. They've been back and forth for dinners, card games and coffee. This would have been a tough one. Not, perhaps as tough as telling us, but still hard to do.

I think, and Gail agrees, having members of the extended family know about the cancer will be more support for Mom and Dad. At the very least it will be less tiring for Mom and Dad to not feel they have to put up a good front and pretend everything is normal. Word will spread through the family now. When I first heard about Dad's cancer I thought if I didn't tell anybody it wouldn't be real. Then, our family spent time together and talked about Dad's cancer but somehow it was comforting being the only ones who knew. Now, all of our family will know and soon the community will find out. That will make it very real. Once this news becomes public I feel a bit like our private time will be over and Dad's cancer will be discussed in general terms much like the day's weather report. Dad is very well known in our little community and I have to expect the residents will be shocked and concerned. I just feel as though having people know will be as exhausting as keeping it quiet. Now, we handle ourselves in ways which protect or boost Dad and Mom's spirits. Soon we will have to display our strength in public. We will have to deal with not only our emotions but soon there will be questions by well-meaning people.

### Tuesday, May 24, 2005

*We* had a good weekend. Ron and I accomplished so many things and I feel good about what we did. Ron washed our front windows inside and out and I cleaned kitchen cupboards and the bathroom cabinets. I tackled the headboard on our bed and got all the books and papers put away. Now we can sleep without fear of being buried under an avalanche of paper! I shopped, baked, cooked a turkey and got the laundry caught up. I read, slept and we made a couple of trips to the cottage to finish raking the leaves.

Ron has been so attentive since we found out about Dad. He has always put the boys and me first but now it is much more. I can't really describe what is different except there is definitely a deeper communication between us. He knows my pain. He knows how much I adore my Dad and how heart broken I am that Dad has to go through this.

We spoke to Mom and Dad on Sunday as per usual. They sounded good and were finding things to keep them busy. Mom sounded really "up" for our annual Mother/Daughter Weekend. She felt things had unfolded in such a way that Dad will be fine on his own and she will be able to relax and enjoy the time away. Gail called me on Monday to say Mom really wanted to go and we have decided to make it happen. She has been living with this nightmare for several months and a brief "time out" maybe what she needs to recharge before Dad's chemotherapy treatments begin. Also, depending on how severe Dad's side effects are from his treatments she may not have another opportunity to get away for awhile. Dad really wants us to continue with our plans. Our Mother/Daughter Weekends have always been a source of pride for Dad. He enjoys knowing we want to be together and don't just talk about it. We actually dedicate time for that purpose. So, we have decided to make it a good weekend and will try to keep the conversation "disease free". Ron wants to go to Dad's and hang-out with him for the weekend but we're going to leave that up to Dad. He may need a weekend on his own, too.

Mom told Gail that Dad has been so strong throughout all of this. He hasn't broken down once. Dad has always been able to reach deep down inside himself and pull strength from his reserves. He has always been able to control his emotions and has been strong regardless of the situation. He told Mom it hurts him to see her or one of us upset. His remarkable faith gives him strength. I hope he isn't in denial or isn't keeping his feelings bottled up which will be hard on his health. But, somehow, I feel what we see is what it really is. Our next job is to prepare to do battle. Our greatest task will be to show Dad we are strong, too, and he has raised three women who will be able to deal with whatever life hands us and will be there for Mom, as well.

I've been doing a lot of reading on the subject of nutrition to fight cancer and to ward off the effects of chemotherapy and radiation. I'm reading about weight loss and how to maintain muscle mass. I also have learned the importance of aromatherapy to help with nausea and induce relaxation and sleep. There are certain smells which help with headaches and help to alleviate mild depression. Color is also very powerful and helps calm or uplift. I want to learn more about keeping Dad comfortable while going through all of this. The medical part I'll leave to the doctors, Cathy and Gail. Mom and I will focus on homeopathic treatments. Laughter is a big part of fighting this disease and so is faith. He has a great sense of humor and his faith is very deep. We'll supplement the laughter with old half-hour situation comedies like *The Beverley Hillbillies* and *Andy Griffith* that we can buy on VHS or DVD. We've always had a great relationship and Dad is very secure of his place in our hearts and lives. We'll just circle the wagons a bit closer to get through this next stage of "life with cancer".

Ron told his Dad a couple of days ago about Dad's cancer. He didn't tell me how Allie reacted but I'm certain he was upset.

Dr. Reid, thoracic surgeon, has ordered one more test to conclusively rule out surgery and after that test is over Dad will have his appointment with his oncologist to set up chemotherapy and radiation schedules. I would like to see him before he starts his treatments. While I know he has cancer I'd like to spend a 'normal' weekend with him. The last weekend we were down he was in such pain with the kidney stone and soon he will start the treatments and we don't know what side effects they will have for him. The last time I saw him feeling well was as they walked away from me at the airport in Panama the end of February. Selfishly, I need a normal weekend with my Dad.

I talked to Cathy this morning just to touch base. I hadn't been talking to her in a week. I've tried calling a few times but the line was busy when I called. She sounded good and busy with her spring cleaning. She was talking about painting their livingroom and cleaning a few more cupboards.

Cathy and I seem to be on the same page regarding supplementary therapies to help Dad fight the cancer. I mentioned the "wasting" which occurs due to lack of appetite or the presence of cancer. She had read something similar. I'll pack a small care package of things I've been reading as well as the tonic we've read about which is great for building the immune system. I asked her to ask the oncologist about the wasting and about sugar feeding the cancer cells. Anything we can do in conjunction with conventional medicine needs to be done. We need to be vigilant in our fight. All ammunition available is worth our investigation.

It was good talking to Cathy and we hung up with promises for a great weekend in Oshawa.

Just after Dad was diagnosed our good friend, Linda, sent me a yellow rubber bracelet which says "Live Strong." The bracelet is sold by the *Lance Armstrong Foundation* in support of cancer research. Brandon saw it when the package arrived and has worn it everyday since. It is a silent recognition of Grandpa's fight and I'm so proud of his quiet support. I have always said he is like Grandpa in many ways but I also see a lot of Ron in him. He doesn't say much but you just know he is there for you.

## Thursday, May 26, 2005

*It's* been one month since I first heard the doctors felt Dad had lung cancer. I think I've gotten over my initial shock and I'm starting to cope better than a month ago. My head and my heart have been in a constant tug-of-war with my reactions. My head wants me to be ruled by my intelligence; to be brave, practical and reliable. My heart wants me to be ruled by my emotions; to cry, relive my memories and admit how scared I am. All the pep talks I've had with myself have really only been my head trying to convince my heart that I have nothing to fear; that the natural order of life is being followed and I should just accept it. In this past month I have learned our minds, bodies and our emotions must take their own time to accept such devastating news. The process can't be hurried along by brave little speeches. The head is probably the quickest to accept. It is our hearts and our bodies which require extra time and I am learning that both will tell me what is needed if only I take the time to listen.

I keep wondering what is going through Dad's mind. If my sisters and I, and Mom when she has a chance, are experiencing all the same waves of emotions and fears then what must Dad be feeling? There must be a struggle going on inside of him. He loves life. He loves us. He is committed to the fight but there must be fear. Dad set the tone for his cancer-challenge the very first day he was given the news. He collected his thoughts, marshalled his emotions and walked into the waiting room and suggested Mom, Dad and my sisters go out for lunch. I really don't think I could have done the same thing. Fear would show in my eyes. So, if he's prepared to be brave for us then, as hard as we may find it, we need to be brave for Dad.

## Tuesday, May 31, 2005

*Yesterday* was Uncle Art's 74<sup>th</sup> birthday. Mom and Dad called him in the morning to sing Happy Birthday. I had sent a card last week. I hope it arrived in time for his special day.

Mom, Cathy, Gail and I met in Oshawa for our Mother/Daughter weekend. We had a really good visit. Our time together was much better than I had expected. Cathy and Gail were really the reason we had such a good time. They clowned and joked around so much they had Mom and I gasping for breath. They really should take their comedy-routine on the road! In private, and for a short time, Mom and I spoke about the initial diagnosis and how we each felt and how Dad was coping but, for the most part, the weekend was kept lighthearted to give Mom a break from the constant strain of living with the knowledge Dad is ill and with the many trips to Kingston to doctors offices. Dad truly is the love of Mom's life and she is certainly his. They have always tried to make the most out of everyday and the need to do that has intensified. I think it was hard for Mom to be away from Dad for even two nights but she really needed to be and it was good for her. Mom called Dad both Friday night and Saturday after we returned from dinner to see how his day had been and how he was feeling.

Dad had sent along a care-package with Mom that he had prepared himself. In the little cooler were tiny bottles of our favorite beverages … Mom received rum and a can of coke, I was sent a scotch, Gail was sent a beer and a small can of clam and tomato juice and Cathy found a wine cooler. The first round of drinks was on Dad!

Dad has an appointment at 9:15 on Thursday morning (June 2) for a test although I can't remember the test's purpose. The results will be ready on Friday (June 3) at 11:15am. I just want them to start treating this insidious thing which is growing inside him. Currently I feel like we are wasting precious time.

Gail graduates from Queen's University on Thursday afternoon. Mom and Dad are so proud. Mom has mentioned that she wanted Gail to compose a little something to put in the local paper with her graduation picture. She deserves to be recognized and I agree. I won't be attending the ceremony because of distance but I will certainly be thinking about her around 2:30pm. Cathy is bringing Dad and Mom in because Dad has his appointment in the morning and they'll all go to the commencement in the afternoon. They will meet Rob at the Jock Hardy Arena where the graduation exercises will take place. What a wonderful day! Gail, unfortunately, has regrets. She feels she sacrificed the past four years worth of weekends studying when she should have been spending time in Sharbot Lake with Mom and Dad. I disagree strongly. Dad would never feel that way nor would he want her to feel her accomplishment is a trade off between her future and spending time with him. Education has always been important to Dad and he encouraged and supported Gail every step of the way.

### Thursday, June 2, 2005

*Two* things happened today. First, Dad had an appointment at 8:15am this morning in Kingston. The surgeon had ordered this test to measure the individual lung capacity and see for sure if surgery is or isn't an option although he feels strongly that it isn't an option. Tests results will be discussed with Mom, Dad and Cathy at 11:15am tomorrow morning.

After the test they went to Gail's for lunch and to rest before Gail's graduation from Queens University took place at 2:30pm. I called Gail's house around 12:30pm and had a chance to talk to everyone. It feels so weird not being there physically to help her celebrate. I feel like our family has so few moments to celebrate left that I should be with them. Tickets were not plentiful and given the number of trips we expect to be making it just didn't seem like the right time to head to Kingston.

After the ceremony they took lots of pictures and then went back to Gail's for drinks around the pool. That's where they gave Gail her presents. She got a kick out of the book the boys bought her … *The Little Engine That Could.*

Mom and Dad called when they got home to tell me all about the day. They were so proud of Gail and happy to be apart of her celebration. Gail called after I talked to Mom and Dad. Like them, she was happy but tired.

We know many of the larger, extended-family has now heard about Dad's illness. Two cousins e-mailed Cathy to get particulars since they didn't feel comfortable repeating such news without knowing the facts. Cathy forwarded the e-mail to Gail and me. We all appreciated their kind words, their offer of support and their respect for our privacy.

## Friday, June 3

*Dad's* at the doctor's office as I write this. I wonder what the test revealed. Personally, I think removing his lung would be an experimental option since the doctors were so certain the surgery wouldn't allow for a good quality of life post-operative and is extremely dangerous to perform. I'd rather they start treatment to shrink the tumor and buy him some time with some quality of life. I just want them to do something which helps my Dad. Curing him doesn't seem to be possible but helping him to breathe easier and enjoy what time we do have seems an achievable goal.

Gail said she'd e-mail when she heard from Mom and Dad. Dad said he'd send me a note when they got home. He didn't imagine they'd be very late since they wanted to get Cathy home as this evening is the Sharbot Lake High School's spring prom and Lindsay and Bradley would be busy getting ready.

---

Subject: Test
Date:    2005 Jun 03—16:12
From:    Harold Clark
To:      Susan Arnold

Hi, Susan;

Just a quick note in another nice day. We got home from Kingston a little after 3pm. Our meeting with the thoracic surgeon went from 11 am to about 11:45 am. He laid the facts on the table. His assistant, Dr Jones, was also present.

First, he was greatly surprised at the results of my tests yesterday. They showed my lung capacity being 67% for the right lung and 32% for the left one. Normal capacity for these are 55% for the right and 45% for the left. So, you see, the right lung has increased its capacity during this episode.

Second, the risk is high at my age with about a 50% cure (with chemo/radiation it would be 30% cure with a potential life span of about 5 years).

The decision is now up to me and the family … surgery verses treatment. We have an open time frame as to when to advise him of our decision. Our first step will be to discuss this with Dr. Bell and then proceed one step at a time.

We will talk with you about this over the weekend at the farm. Have a good day and say "Hi" to all.

Love Dad and Mom

## Monday, June 6, 2005

---

Subject: Gail Graduation
Date:    2005 Jun 06—19:40
From:    Gail Clark
To:      Harold Clark, Susan Arnold, Cathy Fox

Hi, Mom and Dad, Cathy and Susan,

I'm sending along one picture from my graduation. I'll put the others on CD for you. It seems surreal that four years of study are finished … but it was worth it!

**While the words of the Chancellor, as he tapped me on the shoulder, "rise, Bachelor of Arts" are etched in my memory as a moment of pride, the love of my family is treasured in my heart and is the foundation of my past, present and future.**

**Thank all for your gifts, recognition and sharing my special day.**

**Love Always,**

**Gail, B.A**


I'm terrified I may not be able to be as supportive regarding Dad's surgery as I should or want to be. Ultimately, as Ron says, and I agree, it is Dad's decision and we have to support whatever he decides.

One thing this entire journey, that we so abruptly began on April 26th, has taught me is the depth of my love for each of my family, my ability to pretend things are fine when I am in public, how very much I still rely on my Dad for his advice, support, guidance and friendship, and despite all of this how child-like and fragile I really feel. I seem to have stopped thinking and rely more on Ron then ever before to make the smallest decisions. I used to say I was a lot stronger than people realized. I always felt I could rise to any occasion and carry whoever else needed to be carried along as well. Now I realize I'm not as strong in some areas as I thought I was but I'm stronger in surprising ways. I'm strong when it counts. I think this journey will teach me a lot about who I am and what I'm capable of doing.

Apparently, Dad and Mom are going to Dr Bell's to talk to him about the surgery and then, when the decision is final, surgery will be set up very quickly ... within four weeks. I feel in my heart Dad has already made the decision. Included in his thought process, I'm sure, will be to spare himself from being a respiratory invalid and to spare us from watching him deteriorate. Dad feels strongly that he has lived a very full life and has been extremely blessed in many ways. He is ready to take this gamble. If he lives and the surgery is a success then he will consider the time a bonus. If he doesn't make it through the surgery he figures it will just be his time to leave this earth and he is prepared to go. As a child in an adults' body I find it extremely hard to think like that although I am old enough to understand that this is life's cycle. Acceptance is the only way we can get through this. We just have to accept whatever decision and the results which will accompany it.

The roller coaster we are on is so unpredictable that it is, in its own weird way, very predictable. I told Ron that I felt I could play ostrich for a few more years and not have to deal with this yet. I didn't know Dad was seriously considering the surgery. I had lulled myself into pretending Dad's cancer was like my arthritis ... there, but manageable. Stupid, to be sure, but something I desperately needed to believe. The very next morning when I spoke to Mom and Dad it suddenly hit me what Dad was considering and everything that his decision could mean to him and our family ... positively and negatively. So, in less than twelve hours I went from a false sense of calm to feeling the cold grip of fear settling in my stomach, once again, like a flopping fish.

When I spoke to Cathy, she seemed optimistic about the possibility of surgery.
Cathy also mentioned that Gail's Rob had bad news of his own. His father was re-diagnosed with lung cancer thirteen years after his ini-

tial battle. The news didn't sound encouraging. Malcolm has just turned sixty-eight years-old.

## Tuesday, June 7, 2005

*I* just received an e-mail from Gail. She wrote to tell me to hang in. She was afraid, too, but she has been reading a lot of studies and articles about total lung resection on patients over seventy years-old and the predicting of pre/post operative lung-function. What she wrote was optimistic and encouraging to view credible statistics from studies which have been conducted all over the world, and as recent as March of this year. Apparently age is not the risk factor. The three top risk factors are current dependency on others for basic daily activities, reduced mental capacity or dementia and other medical problems such as diabetes and obesity. Dad has none of these. His cancer team seems to feel, based on all his test results that he is a good candidate for the surgery.

Gail ended her e-mail, "I believe that ultimately it's Dad's choice, and whatever decision he makes he has to believe it is the right decision whole-heartedly and we have to be behind him 100%. Even if the worst were to happen and Dad died during the surgery, I believe Dad's feeling is that the same Power that has guided him to choose would be the same Power that guides the outcome. I'm scared too, but I don't want our fears to hold Dad back from what he feels is best for him. His gut instinct hasn't failed him yet. Hang in, Sue. I'm looking forward to seeing you and your family, too. I think this weekend will be profoundly meaningful in the terms of the power of family; our family."

She is so right and I agree whole heartedly. Still, I can't deny anything she has said and I just have to get my thoughts together and my fears under control. I know I can do that without falling to pieces publicly but I really can't determine how well I will be privately if the worst were to happen.

Dad just e-mailed to tell me Dr. Bell had called the house last night and had a lengthy discussion with Mom and Dad over the phone. Dr Bell felt the surgery was a good idea. He said age isn't a factor but the age of the body is; which means that some people are old at fifty because of certain conditions. Aside from Dad's diseased lung he has none of the conditions normally associated with aging. He told Dad the lung would compensate and, much like an athlete, it would increase its capacity if it is exercised and strengthened. Dad said he and Mom were leaning strongly towards the surgery and he would like to have it done as soon as possible.... first part of July if he could be scheduled. He also asked for my honest opinion. Panic! What do I tell him?

---

**Subject: Re: Good Morning**
**Date:    2005 Jun 07—3:47**
**From:   Susan Arnold**
**To:      Harold Clark**

**Hi, Dad;**

**I'm so glad you had a chance to talk to Dr. Bell. You asked for my honest opinion. Really, Dad, my opinion doesn't matter. You have to be 100% convinced surgery is the route you want to go. Your gut instinct and your faith will guide you just as it has guided you every day of your life. However, my feelings are these:**

1. **Cathy seemed very positive about what Dr. Reid and Dr. Jones said to you at your appointment on Friday. He told you at the very beginning he wouldn't operate if he thought it was too risky or your quality and**

life expectancy wouldn't improve, He seems to feel very strongly after your last test that you are a good candidate.

2. Dr. Bell seems to feel, judging from your conversation last night, that it is the best option.

3. Gail's research indicates surgery is a successful option

4. You are physically healthy. No conditions normally associated with aging. I take more medication than you do!

5. You are mentally determined. I believe in the power of positive thinking.

6. We have been very blessed throughout our lives and faith does work miracles.

Dad, for our entire life you have always put the needs and feelings of our family into your decision making. I am begging you, Dad, please put yourself first and make the decision you think is right for you. Whatever you choose I am behind you 100% and so will the rest of the family.

I love you.

Susan

I sure hope my words helped. I think I was just restating the obvious and he will make the final decision.

## Wednesday, June 8, 2005

---

Subject: Re: Hi
Date:    2005 Jun 08—10:44
From:    Gail Clark
To:      Susan Arnold

Hi, Sue!

How right you are about finding the joy in each day … or at least giving yourself time and space to look for it. I also think you're right on the money when you say we'll discover things about ourselves or confirm things we never think about. I guess I've discovered my faith is alive and well when I thought it had faded. I also confirm the knowledge that when our family pulls together the force is truly awesome!

I just got back from an interview for Project Leader. The message light on my phone was flashing when I sat down at my desk. It was Dad calling to see how the interview went! He never forgets! The message said they are on their way to the farm and that he'd call me tonight when they're back.

I think we're planning to come to the farm Saturday morning. I want to make the pasta salad and clean the vegetables for the veggie platter on Friday night so I don't have to do it when I get there.

I'll talk to you soon.

Love Gail

*Gail* phoned last night and we spoke for well over an hour. Dad had canvassed all three of us for our honest opinions. He had told Gail that, unless I had any strong feelings against surgery, he wanted to get it organized as soon as possible. We are both of the opinion that, as soon as Dad received my e-mail, he was on the phone with the surgeon's office.

We discussed our fears and everything Dad is and stands for and believes in. We have concluded, once the emotion is taken out of the equation, that surgery is the best option regardless of what the outcome is. Either way, Dad will not have to suffer through the agony of a slow deterioration. This is his decision and we all know it is his best shot.

I feel time slipping away from me this year. I live from one of Dad's appointment dates to the next. It seems like yesterday since I found out about the cancer but it was the end of April now it is the 8th of June.

Last weekend Ron and I went out a couple of times and really enjoyed ourselves which helped take the pressure off everything which has been going on. We attended the Blackfly Gala on Friday evening which was a beautiful Italian buffet and entertainment. The next evening we went to a card party at the home of some friends. I'm not much of a card-shark but the evening was a lot of fun.

Friends of ours have been talking about going to dinner. We need to socialize to help de-stress. For so many years we have focused on the children and their events and activities. Now I think we need to start cultivating our own calendar of events. Since we are home next weekend maybe we should think about going out for dinner then.

It seems sort of surreal to be planning a social life and a summer when my Dad's life is so tenuous. However, I was raised with my Dad's principles. Life is for the living and "all work and no play makes Jack a dull boy." It really isn't the fun or the activity, Dad wants all of us to have a support system in life which extends beyond the family.

I want to make a real effort at increasing the "joy" factor in my life. Joy doesn't require money but it does require imagination and effort (mental and physical). While the boys were little I would make pancake breakfasts outside before school, we planted tomatoes and dug for buried treasure. Now, it is a little harder to come up with everyday things that the boys enjoy but I still try to make an effort and set an example of joyful living. My Dad has always had an interest in life and is passionate about living. I had the example set for me and I need to make sure I don't slack-off on my duty as a parent. Joy can be found in a cup of freshly-brewed coffee sipped on the deck at the cottage in the quiet of the early morning. Joy can be a sunset kayak ride with Ron. Joy can take many forms and I must put forth an effort to embrace them all.

Each of the boys seems to have their own personal way of supporting Grandpa. Greg is trying extra hard in math and plans to take his most recent good test papers to the farm, in Arden, to show Grandpa. Brandon has been wearing his yellow Lance Armstrong "Live Strong" bracelet to support cancer patients and research. He hasn't taken it off since he received it from Aunt Linda early in May. Ron's support comes in many forms. He chats on the telephone to Dad and Mom, extra hugs for me and he is always finding ways of bringing a smile to my face or making life a little less stressful. Ron has suggested he go to Sharbot Lake to help Mom and Dad as long as I can cope with things here. He is planning to be with me, in Kingston, when Dad's surgery is taking place. His support, like his love, is unfailing. I've always loved him with all my heart but lately the feeling has actually deepened and that surprises me as I felt I couldn't love him more than I did. He is one of the blessings God has provided me and my family. He sent Ron to me and then added our two sons.

---

**Subject: Re: Good Morning!**
**Date:    2005 Jun 08—13:22**
**From:   Harold Clark**
**To:       Susan Arnold**

Hi, Susan;

We're getting along fine. Mom is starting to pack some things for the weekend. If it doesn't rain we are taking Bradley with us to the farm. He can cut the grass and trim up-we can unpack the things Mom has for the first load. It will be that much less to remember on Friday.

Regarding your e-mail yesterday. I/we really appreciated hearing your thoughts. You guessed right. At 11 am today I called Dr. Reid's office to advise him of my decision to go through with the surgery. I am now awaiting a return call to confirm the formalities for pre op. We will keep you informed.

Art and Sue dropped in last Friday evening but we were out at Cathy and Steve's watching the kids get ready for the formal. Mom called them later. They are doing fine.

Not much else going on here. We're anxious to see you all over the weekend.

Take care. Have a good day and we'll talk soon.

Love Mom and Dad

**3pm**

So, a decision has been made and I'm back to the waves of emotions I went through when we first heard about this in April. Given how quickly things have happened I am certain we will have a date we can plan around by the end of the week. Practical has to overtake emotional now the decision has been made. Things must get organized here at the office to allow me to be away without concern that I've forgotten something important.

My mind is just a flurry of thoughts ... from one extreme to the other. I have the same sort of a feeling I used to have as a student facing an exam or, now, as the Treasurer, awaiting the annual audit. The date will be circled on the calendar and it will come and go like any other day. The difference with this date, when we get it, is it won't be "any other day." This will be a day like no other in my entire life. I can't even imagine those hours leading up to the surgery or the hours while he is being operated on. It might just as well be me on the operating table with Dad. We are definitely all tied to one another.

---

**Subject: Dad**
**Date:    2005 Jun 08—3:35**
**From:   Susan Arnold**
**To:      Gail Clark**

Just a quick heads up. I asked Dad outright this morning if he had already spoken to Dr. Reid's office and he confirmed he had at 11 am today.

Just cook the pasta and we'll mix it up at the farm. Regarding the vegetables; bring them along. It will give us something to do to keep our emotions in check. Good luck on the job interview.

See you soon,

Susan

---

Subject: Re: Dad
Date:    2005 Jun 08—15:59
From:   Gail Clark
To:      Susan Arnold

Thanks for the advance notice ... I'm coming Friday for sure. Dad must be exhausted from wrestling with the decision but most likely he's also relieved that it's done. I wonder when the surgery will be? I hope it is after their anniversary.

Later,

Gail

## Friday, June 10, 2005

---

Subject: Re: Good Morning!
Date:    2005 Jun 10—12:09
From:   Gail Clark
To:      Susan Arnold

Hi, Sue;

Just got back from coffee with Mom and Dad after the consultation with Dr. Reid. I really think Dad is in good hands with Dr. Reid. You can tell he's confident about what he does but not in a proud, boastful way; more like a capable, skilled way.

He recapped the events leading up to Dad's decision for surgery and expressed his confidence in the above average capacity in his right lung. He said Dad should expect a complete removal of the left lung (given the slight chance that he could save any part). He anticipates Dad will not require oxygen assisted breathing after release from hospital. During recuperation, if Dad feels any difficulty in breathing he will be referred to the respiratory rehab unit at St. Mary's but he doesn't foresee that based on preoperative lung capacity. Dad can expect to feel a perceived decline in oxygen level for approximately three months while he heals and the other lungs gets back up to normal functioning ... just like athletic conditioning where you feel worse before you feel better.

Otherwise, he mentioned the procedure will be done through Dad's ribs; they'll cut the muscle between the ribs. He said it is not uncommon to break a rib during the operation particularly with elderly patients. This is normal regardless of osteoporosis or not. The only surprise is that the surgery may happen sooner rather than later. Dr. Reid said they will do the preoperative assessment approximately one week before surgery. Dad should expect a call to arrange that next week and the surgery will probably be done by the end of June or the first week of July. Dad's good with that, though, ... he said, "the sooner the better"!

Anyway, Sue, Dad is totally ready for this ... you can see it in his eyes that he believes it's the right choice and he has complete confidence in Dr. Reid's ability. I do, too. "All for one and one for all!

As for Rob's Dad, there's no new news yet ... he's scheduled for a needle biopsy on the 17th and I guess he'll get more direction after that.

**Anyway, Sue, I'd better go.**

**See ya,**

**Love Gail**


***There*** is one date I hope and pray it isn't … actually two dates. The first would be their forty-ninth wedding anniversary on June 30 and the second is June 27, the anniversary of the passing of his only sibling; his younger sister. She was a kindergarten teacher who died in a car accident when a drunk seventeen year-old ran a stop sign on the last day of school. She was thirty-four years-old.

We're heading to the farm for a weekend with the family. Both Lindsay and Bradley have the weekend off from their part-time jobs so there won't be anyone missing from the group. I'm looking forward to the weekend but I'm also thinking there may be an announcement regarding the farm. The man who has shown an interest has been back to the farm several times and looked through the farm house on his last visit. He'd like to have the deal close as soon as possible. That is far too much pressure and emotional change for me to feel comfortable about but I'll have to go along with whatever Mom and Dad decide.

*Brandon*

*The farm was a special place. It has a lake, lots of forest, sand pits to play around in and all kinds of trails for the four wheelers to go. The farm is at the end of Clark Road and on one part of the farm there is still the log cabin my great-great-grandfather built. It was really fun having the family all stay there for weekends in the summer or in the fall. There were always lots to do at the farm. We would fish, go for* walks, drive the four wheelers everywhere and sit under the pine tree in the afternoons. In the evenings we would go to the old Swimming Hole to clean up and jump off the diving board and then Grandma would have a bonfire ready before we got back. The stars were really bright in the country and we could hear the wolves in the distance and Grandma answering them back. The Whipperwill would call each evening to his mate from one of the trees.

Grandpa would always show us where bears had clawed a tree or deer had chewed up a bush. That was cool to see. Sometimes he'd take us to places on the farm where he had gone to get the cattle when he was just a boy or he'd show us the spring where he'd bring back his family's water.

### Tuesday, June 14, 2005

---

Subject: Weekend!!!
Date:    2005 Jun 13—14:46
From:    Harold Clark
To:      Susan Arnold, Cathy Fox, Gail Clark

Hi, All;

Mom and I want to thank everyone for another great weekend at the farm. The effort of each certainly rounded out the stay and contributed to the usual good laughs and jokes that make a good tonic for all. We enjoyed a warm welcome weather-wise and the rain stayed away and let us play. It's another one to remember. Again ... many thanks!

Love Mom and Dad

We had a great weekend. Dad looked a little frail, and didn't move around much due to the heat and extreme humidity but was in great spirits and looked quite confident about his decision. We didn't discuss it much but touched on it in other ways. Dad told us Mom had asked him to tell the man interested in purchasing the farm that they wouldn't be selling for awhile. Dad was having surgery and the family just isn't prepared to handle the emotional break a sale would mean as well as the work of preparing for an auction. Good for Mom! Dad seemed relieved as well. There is no point selling to the first bidder because Dad's health is questionable.

Dad did tell each of us to look around the farm and see if there was anything we wanted as a memento. I selected the rocking chair from behind the kitchen door and the small, ornamental elephant that has stood on a corner-shelf in the dining room for as long as I can remember. Brandon would like the farm! He even wondered if Grandpa would sell it to him. He has almost $500 saved! Bless his heart.

As I wandered through the old farmhouse I saw, in my mind's eye, the many memories I had of my grandparents and other relatives who had visited. I remembered my sisters and I would pretend the pull-down door of the dining room china hutch was our oven and we would "bake" up a storm while the adults talked in the kitchen. I remembered sitting on my Grandfather's knee in the rocking chair and feeling so special perched where I had a bird's eye-view of everything going on around me.

In the United States between the 1890's and the 1930's a new style of house plan became very popular. The home was a one-storey design, a bungalow, and most of the new homes being built used this new style. The plan didn't catch on in Canada until after World

War II and during the 1950's and 1960's bungalows were built across the country. Their compact layout allowed the homemakers of the day to carryout her various tasks with more efficiency and saved her steps while doing so.

The farmhouse had been built by my grandparents when they had returned to Canada in 1932 after living for nine years in Watertown, New York during the Depression Years. They had seen this new style of home and appreciated the benefits that would come from building a bungalow instead of the usual two-storey farmhouse. And so, twenty years before the bungalow became a common and fashionable building-style in Canada, my grandparents were constructing their new home on a piece of property purchased from my great-grandfather. Residents from all over the county came to look at the structure and marvel at the modern design where all the living space was on one floor.

Several times during the weekend Dad gave instructions about what items were stored in the barn and in the henhouse and what value each item was perceived to have in case we needed to organize a sale. He kept it very upbeat but he was preparing us in case things didn't go well with his surgery. I had a couple of difficult moments. Especially when I would listen to Dad tell stories about the farm or his childhood. They are stories I've heard many times but somehow never remember and never tire of hearing again.

Aside from the high humidity that made it difficult to sleep, the weekend went by with the usual good times and laughter, but there was a palpable realization of what this weekend may represent. The rain stayed away and let us get out and enjoy the farm. Leaving was easier because we are planning to come down in two weeks.

I hope to put flowers in the planter at the front of our house this evening. I think the threat of frost has past and the house can use the color. Ron is supposed to whipper-snip the yard at the house and the cottage this afternoon. I also want to clean the bar area of the Rec room. I'd like to get as much done as I can before the weekend and then, spend time at the cottage cleaning inside it and the bunkhouse. I'd like everything to be ready for us to move into for the summer. Our target date is June 30.

Everyone I talk to is so positive about the surgery and speaks as if it is a simple operation. I'm still very afraid but I know this is the best option. I also feel like a bit of a liar. I told Dad, if he decided to go ahead with the surgery, I'd support him 100%. I will support his decision. That much is true but I don't feel this surgery is his best option. I hope I'm proven wrong. If things go according to plan then Dad will no longer have the cancer tumor and his cough will be gone and he will have a chance at a normal life. I'm just not ready to lose my Dad yet and part of me hasn't really accepted that this has happened. The cancer has been growing on his lung while we were in Panama, while we were eating Christmas dinner, when they drove up to celebrate Ron's birthday, while they visited us at the cottage. It was like a horrible monster; waiting, silently growing and gaining strength. In my head, I see him coming through the surgery and then, after a few months, being as good as new. Then, when I least expect it I become consumed with fear.

**Monday, June 20, 2005**

---

**Subject: Report**
**Date:    2005 Jun 20—12:01**

From:   Harold Clark
To:     Susan Arnold, Cathy Fox, Gail Clark

Hi,

Just so I can't be blamed for not letting everyone know….
I have had a call from Dr. Reid's office with the following:

1) Be at the Hotel Dieu Hospital at 10 am June 23 for pre admission testing

2) I will undergo surgery Monday, June 27. I'll receive final details on admission Sunday afternoon.

This is all I know at present but will keep everyone posted as we find out the particulars.

Love, Dad

*Dad* just e-mailed. He has a pre-admissions test on Thursday (June 23) and surgery has been scheduled for Monday, June 27. That's a week from today! That's a week from right now! Seeing the date in print makes it all too real! How the hell did we get here? I'm not ready for this!

I can't really get my mind around things. I feel like I've gone back in time to the end of April when this nightmare started. The lump has returned to my throat. I've learned to function by pretending everything is fine but inside I'm a mess. My whole world is rocking. Dad has always been the pin which secures our family. I can't possibly imagine life any other way than how it is now. The way it has always been. Ron knows the feeling. His life changed so suddenly when his mom died. Her death was quick and it was all over before the shock wore off. We've had time to think about what might happen and pray to the Heavens it doesn't.

## Tuesday, June 21, 2005

*Today* is the first day of summer; the longest day of the year. I have a feeling that, for this year, the longest day will be June 27.

## Wednesday, June 22, 2005

---

**Subject: Dad's Surgery**
**Date:**    2005 Jun 22—15:08
**From:**    Gail Clark
**To:**      Susan Arnold

I imagine this is stupid to ask but are you coming home for Dad's surgery? You're welcome to stay with me and I'm going to ask mom if she wanted to be in Kingston, too. I have two extra bedrooms and they might as well be used. You can think about it and let me know.

Love,

Gail

---

Gail and I spoke at length last night. She had sent me the bus schedule from Kingston to North Bay. She knows Ron is coming with me and will stay for a couple of days after the surgery but she felt, if I could arrange it, perhaps I could stay down a bit longer and return via the bus. I said it was definitely something to keep in mind. I don't want to make any plans right now. I prefer to see how things unfold and make our plans as we need.

My biggest concern at the moment is the boys. Ron and I have discussed whether or not to bring the boys to the hospital for the surgery. We agree having them at home will be better for them and, Brandon will graduate from Grade Six on the same day as the surgery. They don't want to leave their own home for four or more days to stay with relatives and I want them to be together. Ron thinks they would be fine on their own if their cousin, Chad, were to come to the house to stay at night. Uncle Steve Arnold would check-in on them and Uncle Perry Arnold is around the corner on the next street if they needed help. I know, with rules, they would be OK but I don't know if this is the time to start leaving them. We've never left them alone overnight before and I worry so much when they are away from me. I just don't feel comfortable with this scenario. Our boys tell me they would do the laundry and run the dishwasher and keep things tidy. That's nice to hear but I'm more concerned with a four-wheeler ride which upsets or a stove left on. What is the guideline? When are they old enough for me to trust they will be safe if they are left alone and when am I giving them too much freedom? I don't want to put them in a position they aren't capable of dealing with. I want them with us but the hospital is just not the right place for them to be. I really don't know what to do. I'm very worried about leaving the boys and perhaps my worry is making the problem bigger then it is. Chad is nineteen. Our boys are twelve and almost fifteen. I'll defer to Ron's judgment. He would never suggest something he didn't truly believe they could handle.

Uncle Steve Arnold and Greg will attend Brandon's graduation in our place. Casper, our four year-old Labrador has been booked into the kennel in North Bay so he won't be an added responsibility for the boys while we are gone.

Dad is still sounding very upbeat. The stress is starting to sound in Mom's voice but she is doing really well given the fact that she has been living with this for longer than we have.

I really haven't eaten much since Monday. I've had yogurt, bananas, salads and a sandwich but I just don't feel hungry and nothing really appeals to me.

## Saturday, June 25, 2005

*Ron* and I left for Sharbot Lake around 11am. I'm feeling uneasy and can't find anything concrete to blame.

We arrived at Sharbot Lake to find tensions running very high. Dad was trying hard to appear as though he wasn't nervous or stressed and failing miserably since small little things suddenly became gigantic problems. Ron and I decided to take them for a drive to Cathy's after dinner to help alleviate the stress.

Everyone was ready for an early night.

## Sunday, June 26, 2007

*Mom* and Dad have been receiving a lot of visitors over the past week. In an eerie way it felt like a wake before a death. I can't imagine how Dad must have been feeling.

The churches in Sharbot Lake were all going to announce Dad's cancer and his scheduled surgery at the various services. Cathy and Steve had invited us to breakfast on Sunday morning and Mom and Dad didn't try to be stoic and stay at home. We needed our privacy and felt some friends may want to drop-in at Mom and Dad's house and wish him well when they heard his news. With the atmosphere so tension-filled we thought it best to simply not be at home. Mom and Dad willingly went and we had a pleasant time. Cathy cooked bacon and eggs and then we sat out on their deck and visited. I went for a swim in the pool and by 1:30pm we headed back to Mom and Dad's.

We felt we should leave for Gail's house in Kingston at a fairly decent hour to allow Mom and Dad time to prepare for the next day. Leaving was very hard. We tried to keep it light and short.

We joked and bantered as per usual but when I gave Dad a hug and whispered, "I love you," he dissolved in my arms ... for the briefest of moments ... then he recovered and I was left to wonder if it had actually happened. I didn't try to say anything more ... I couldn't since my throat was so constricted. I simply smiled, waved and left. What else could I do?

We arrived at Gail's. Rob was there and the two of them prepared us a wonderful BBQ. We sat around her swimming pool discussing Dad's surgery the next day.

We went to bed early since 4:30am would come quickly.

## Monday, June 27, 2005

*What* a roller coaster of emotion we have experienced today. While we feared the surgery we also felt hope.

I didn't sleep a single wink. I lay awake all night long listening to the sound of the traffic outside on the street in front of Gail's house and the ticking of the alarm clock which was on the tiny table to the left of my head. The alarm was set for 4:30am. At 4am I got up and washed my hair. There was no point trying to sleep for a half hour. Soon Gail, Rob and Ron were up, too.

We left for the hospital at 5:15am planning to get there before Dad. Each of us drove to the hospital lost in our own thoughts.

We arrived in the hospital lobby and not long after Dad, Mom, Cathy, Steve and their kids came in from the parking area. Dad looked tired and pale but maintained his composure when he saw our family's solidarity. I'm sure I would have lost it seeing everyone there to support me.

Dad, Mom and Cathy went up to register and then Cathy came to get us.

Dad was changed into a hospital gown and was waiting in a hospital bed to be wheeled to surgery. We stayed with him until 7:50am when the nurse came to take him to the operating room. He looked so small and fragile in that big hospital bed. In that emotional and highly-charged moment Dad finally broke down which was difficult to see. He was wheeled through the "Restricted. No Admittance" doors and we were left with each other and time.

We suggested to Mom that we should get something to eat in the café since Dad had been very concerned that we hadn't eaten yet. Dad must carry the Italian gene! While we were there Mom and Dad's minister, Patsy, arrived and joined us for a coffee.

We received word the surgery was progressing well in the operating room and Dad's operation should be completed by 10am. We were so relieved. Ron and I decided to get out of the hospital and take a walk by Lake Ontario.

At 9:20am we headed back inside to see if there was any further word from surgery. As we came down the hospital hallway I saw my entire family being ushered into a little room and someone had their arms around Mom. Something was very wrong! I felt panic take hold and I had the sensation of separating from my body and began a spectator-like existence watching my own life as it unfolded. We got to the door and saw everyone crying but nobody said anything. I heard myself repeatedly ask, "What? What?" I felt light-headed as I waited for someone to tell me what was going on. Mom told me to "sit here" and she indicated a spot beside her. Oh, Dear God, has Dad died? Why else would my family be here like this? I *knew* this surgery was a bad idea. Although my eyes were pinned on Mom I felt Ron's hand on my shoulder and I could feel the tears on my face.

Gail was sitting on the other side of Mom, holding both her hands, "It's OK, Susan, he's still alive," she whispered. The relief I felt was immediate and immense. Still, something was very wrong. Gail had a haunted, frightened look in her eyes. I couldn't see Cathy's face. She was sitting, bent over, with her head in her hands. Mom was softly crying. The surgeon had found the family in the waiting room and told them they couldn't take out the lung because they had found more cancer on the lining of the lung and on the inside of his chest. Dr Reid came back to talk to the whole family and explain what this means and to answer any questions we may have had.

As the doctor spoke we were all in shock. I hadn't even considered this possibility. I don't think any of us had. The doctors had been so convinced the cancer was contained on Dad's lung. I had thought about the removal of his lung, the chance that he wouldn't survive the surgery and the complications which could occur after the surgery but this never once crossed my mind. Dad had gone through this invasive surgery and was no further ahead, and was actually behind as he now has to recover from the operation that hadn't achieved what it was intended to achieve. They had opened him up and were preparing to remove the lung when the additional cancer-sites had been discovered. It was a huge disappointment. Knowing the reason for the change of plans was mind-numbing. The realization that Dad still had the cancer we knew about and more we hadn't known about growing inside him and knowing there would be nothing else aside from chemotherapy and radiation to help him only overwhelmed us with emotion. We felt Dad's disappointment keenly. Dad would be expecting to wakeup and be told the lung was gone. We felt fear for all of us as the future suddenly looked so frightening. The room was small and warm and grew warmer by the second. Nobody spoke. Everyone seemed to be struggling with the reality of the situation, and denial, all at the same time. I had to get out of the room. I had to get some air.

As the shock subsided we began to discuss things more rationally and try to make some sense out of everything. Dad was a long time being brought to room 435 on Kidd 4. The doctor spoke with him and told him they hadn't removed the lung and, although Dad was still pretty groggy, he appeared to understand. Despite the disappointment and the effects of his medication he simply said to each of us, "We tried. Now we'll go on to Plan B." He is so factual, so logical and so willing to discuss it without dwelling on the negative. I wish I could be half as strong. I've heard it said that the prospect of dying is harder on the family than the actual patient. Perhaps there is truth to that statement. Dad's first thought has always been to protect us and keep us from being afraid. He is still doing this.

We decided, after visiting with Dad (two at a time) that we should go to Gail's and see if Mom might lie down for a bit of a rest before dinner. I'm not sure how much sleep Mom and Dad had gotten the night before (although they both said they slept not too badly) but we knew their day had started around 3:30am. It was then 4pm. Ron, bless his heart, insisted on staying quietly in Dad's room in case he needed something. We came back to the hospital around 7pm and stayed until visiting hours were over at 8pm.

What a day! We had started out with such high hopes and by the evening they were dashed to smithereens.

### Wednesday, June 29, 2005

*Ron* and I went to the hospital a bit early today. Gail, Mom and Cathy arrived later. Ron is heading back to South River today. As glad as I am that he will be with the boys and will touch base with the store I will really miss him. We've been so connected and he knows when I'm too emotional to speak and steps in to fill the gap until I can speak. He's been my strength and a huge comfort to everyone. He stayed Monday and Tuesday evening with Dad when we left in the afternoon for a rest and our dinner. He needed to be with Dad and felt Dad may need assistance in sitting up to cough and he'd be able to help. Coughing and expelling the mucus in the lungs are vital after surgery to prevent pneumonia. The incision made coughing painful and Dad found if someone firmly pressed a pillow into his side he was able to cough. I was afraid of hurting Dad when I tried to press the pillow into his side but Ron was able to apply just the right amount of pressure.

Ron left Kingston a little before 2pm with promises to call when he reached South River. As he drove away I felt like part of me was leaving.

### Thursday, June 30, 2005

*Today* is Mom and Dad's forty-ninth wedding anniversary. Dad had asked me just before I left yesterday if I would purchase an anniversary card for him to give to Mom. He had tried to get one on Thursday when they had been in for his pre-surgery appointment but Mom seemed determined to stay beside him all day! Dad had such a wonderful day yesterday and, not thinking that things could change so quickly, Cathy, Gail and I decided to make their anniversary special. We brought a lace tablecloth from Gail's along with champagne flutes, non alcoholic champagne; a potted miniature rose and we brought Chinese food. Dad was sleeping when we arrived but we decided to set up anyway. We couldn't have known he had been awake most of the night with pain and had been sick in the morning. We had forgotten, in the excitement of seeing Dad so well, the second day after surgery is usually worse then the first day. He was on intervenes medication to help settle his stomach. He slept most of the day and awoke long enough to have a short visit with us and to give Mom her card. They toasted each other with a glass of the sparkling cider and my sisters and I slipped out of the room to allow them some private time. Mom said our gesture really meant so much to both of them and Dad was so pleased we had made the effort. We just wanted to do what they would normally do … recognize and make their anniversary special.

Gail and Rob took possession of their new twenty-one foot boat today. It has sleeping quarters, a potty and BBQ so it is legally classified as a residence. The timing wasn't great. Gail didn't seem as enthusiastic as she should have felt but they went out on the water-test and seemed impressed with their purchase. I look forward to seeing it and, someday, getting a ride in it.

# _Part Three_

# _Summer 2005_

## Friday, July 1, 2005

*Today* is Canada Day. I borrowed Gail's vehicle and drove over to the bus station to pick up my ticket for tomorrow. I leave Kingston at 7am and arrive, via Ottawa, in North Bay at 3:20pm. It is going to be hard leaving Dad.

He still has some of his tubing in place, and he seems so frail and foggy. I know it is the pain and the medication but it is so hard trying to visualize Dad being strong and healthy again. The staff who worked in his ward have been wonderfully attentive. He has someone checking him constantly and his every want or need is looked after. In fact, they are so attentive Dad feels a little embarrassed by all the fuss. I've heard so many horror stories about lack of staff in hospitals and poor quality nursing in news reports and I can't say we've experienced that at all.

When visiting hours were just about over and I recognized the signs that Mom and Gail were getting ready to leave I began to feel unsure about my decision to leave. Dad wanted me to go back to South River and be with my family and not miss any more work because of him. I'm going just to pacify him. He told me to be good and to have a safe trip home. He asked me to call when I got there so Mom would know I was safe and she could tell him in the morning. The entire time he was speaking I was straightening his bed sheets, tugging them tighter around his middle, rubbing his shoulder and offering him water. I just needed to keep doing for him. I certainly didn't want to dissolve into tears and make this hard for everyone so if I concentrated on a task it kept me from focusing too much on leaving him. I kissed his forehead, told him I loved him and walked out the door.

I did really well! No tears until I got outside his room. Mom and Gail knew I was having a hard time and they allowed me a few moments to collect my thoughts. Gail whispered some encouraging words to me and Mom took my hand as we walked out of the hospital.

## Saturday, July 2, 2005

*It* was an early start. Mom and Gail took me to the bus terminal and stayed until the bus left. At the other end, Ron arrived at the North Bay terminal the same time as the bus. I was so happy to see him! He and the boys had moved us out to the cottage on Friday and soon I would be at our little piece of paradise, too.

## Sunday, July 3, 2005

*Ron* and I called Dad at the hospital at noon as per our usual Sunday routine. Mom answered and told me there was a possibility that Dad would be released in the afternoon. He'd had a pretty good night but was still on oxygen and the nurse wanted to be sure his levels were normal after moving around on his own without the oxygen tube. They removed the oxygen at 11am and promised they'd make a decision by 2pm.

Dad was released with the condition that he would stay in Kingston for the night. That was easy! We had already decided he was spending one or two nights at Gail's. I spoke to him there in the evening and he sounded so much better. The difference was like night and day. Mom sounded better, too. Cathy and Steve came in to stay the night at Gail's. Cathy could check Dad's vitals throughout the night and Steve would drive them all home to Sharbot Lake the next morning if Dad had a good night and felt well. Having his family around has always been the best possible medicine for Dad.

Dad had told Mom there was lots of room in the bed for her to crawl in beside him which would help both of them have a better rest.

I feel more relieved and happy to hear Dad sounding so much stronger.

Ron and I were talking and I told him it wasn't the possibility of losing Dad which upsets me. Ever since I was a little girl I knew there would come a day when I would have to say good-bye to both my parents. It terrified me then and it terrifies me now. What disturbs me so much is the idea that he'll have to suffer and I won't be able to do a damn thing to help him. Watching him deteriorate and slowly suffer will break my heart.

The Eagle Lake Cottage Association took up a collection and had a fireworks display this evening at dusk. Ron, our boys and Casper rode in our boat while friends of ours were in another boat. We tied up the two boats and passed snacks and pop back and forth and had a little visit. Casper wasn't afraid of the noise from the fireworks as they were ignited. In fact, he sat on one of the boat-seats and watched each display intently! The fireworks were spectacular!

Ron woke me up with my morning coffee. He is such a wonderful guy and I'm so lucky to have him in my life. I try never to let a day go by without thinking that and letting him know I love him and appreciate everything he does for our family.

Later, Ron cleaned the gutters at the cottage while I cleaned the wooden lawn furniture. Ron took the boys to hockey in the afternoon and I put some curtains up across the front window. The curtains, toppers really, are a cheery, tropical stripe which matches the cover on the futon and makes the whole place seem happy and shows a bit of the Caribbean influence we have come to love. Brandon looked around the cottage tonight and said, "You know, Mom, our cottage is really colourful." Brandon likes colour and he is pleased with our bright, festive colours.

## Monday, July 4, 2005

*Gail* e-mailed me briefly to let me know that Dad had a good night. Everyone went to bed, at her house, around 10pm and Dad slept well. He was awake to take a painkiller around 2am (not because it was severe but to ward it off) and once to visit the washroom. He was at the breakfast table when Gail left for work and had an orange, tea and toast.

We've decided to give Dad and Mom some space and let them call us rather than making them feel like they live in a glass bowl. They will want to get back into their normal routine and I can't blame them. I was starting to feel at bit like a fish out of water, too.

Ron, Greg and I went for a swim tonight. Casper and Brandon were our lifeguards on the dock. The water was cold at first but it felt refreshing and comfortable soon after getting wet. Ron and Greg washed the kayaks and the two boys went for a little paddle before dark. I like early morning paddles when I'm on my own and the day is filled with possibilities but I love the paddles Ron and I take after dinner when it is just the two of us. We chat about our day and make plans for the future or simply glide along silently together.

## Tuesday, July 5, 2005

*I* sent Dad and Mom an e-mail this morning but so far I haven't received an answer. Once he starts to feel a little more settled I'm sure it won't be long until he pulls the computer out and gets back into our morning routine.

I spoke to Cathy at noon today and she felt Dad was doing pretty well. There have been some phone calls but not as many as I had expected although many people may not realize he is home from the hospital yet.

I've had several people drop into my office to ask after Dad and, while I try not to dwell on it, their concern is very touching. I'm used to having Ron act as my buffer and taking over if he sees me falter. The good wishes and concern for Dad and our family are heart warming and I'm lucky to live in a community so far away from my hometown and yet be surrounded with such caring people. We look for blessings where we can find them and the people in this community can certainly count as a blessing.

## Wednesday, July 6, 2005

*Ron* took Greg to roller hockey in North Bay and when he was leaving he asked if I was planning to call Mom and Dad. I hadn't planned to call but decided maybe I would give them a ring. I hadn't spoken to them since Sunday evening at Gail's. I should have trusted my instincts. Dad's stomach wasn't very good; likely because the painkillers are irritating the stomach lining. Cathy was there with them when I called. Mom said they hadn't slept much the night before as Dad felt sick to his stomach much of the night and most of the day. I wish I hadn't called. I was so happy on Sunday evening to hear him sounding more like himself and less medicated. I've decided, for the time being, when I hear him sounding strong and getting along well I'll wait to hear from them. I'm finding my mood for the day is directly affected by how Dad is. If he's good then I'm good. If he's had a set back then I'm depressed. Dad wouldn't want his medical condition to have that much of an influence on my life and, I suppose, like everything else we've adjusted to, I'll get a handle on this as well. Once he starts chemotherapy his days maybe a mixture of good days and bad days. He'll want to lay low on his bad days and I'll want to play ostrich when I can. I'm sure this isn't a good way of handling it but, until I figure something else out, it's the only way I know.

Dad had a couple of people visit yesterday afternoon and Mom mentioned to them that he tired easily. Nice way of saying, "don't stay too long."

I feel like I'm getting out of my routines since being in Kingston and moving out to the cottage for the summer. I'm not exercising as much as I should, I'm eating more snack foods between meals and more summer "junk" foods for meals and I'm not taking my supplements. I'm just not motivated in the same way as before. Since I found out about Dad's disease I have been to the gym just five times in two months. I have to start taking better care of myself. If anything, staying in good health for both Dad and Mom should make me even more motivated. Starting today I'm going to make an effort to get back into routine. I did pretty well while I was in Kingston; food wise. I made healthy choices and didn't do much snacking in between meals. Perhaps that was the key. What I did eat was prepared and I had choices. Here, I try to find something quick and will settle for what's available even if it isn't healthy. Ron brought home donuts last night. I love donuts! Fortunately, the boys had company staying overnight and they took the donuts out to the bunkhouse for a snack. There probably isn't a crumb left this morning!

---

**Subject: Catching Up**
**Date:    2005 Jul 06—14:34**
**From:   Harold Clark**
**To:     Susan Arnold, Gail Clark**

Hi,

I must confess—I'm lax. Just opened the computer and it looks like I have some work to do. You're both wondering how we are getting along. Well, yesterday was a bit of a down day but today seems a bit better ... as we said earlier, :one day at a time". We have been fortunate so far ... we have had visitors but not so many that it is tiring.

The Women's Institute sent a beautiful blanket and some of the church members have stopped by briefly. So, it's been very good so far.

Mom has done two baskets of strawberries that Cathy and Lindsay picked this morning. She also did her weekly washing in between catering to me. So, you see, we are doing well.

Nothing more to report so I'll scoot ...

Take care and we will talk to you later.

Love Mom and Dad

---

Dad just e-mailed. It was great seeing his name pop up on the screen; like a normal day. He sent it to both Gail and I and it was very brief but still a step in the right direction. He mentions "One day at a time" and indicates he is feeling better today than he did yesterday. It is just so hard to believe we are dealing with this. Dad has never said, but I know, he is disappointed about the way the surgery turned out. He had his hopes set so high that this would be the answer. He had willingly gone into the surgery knowing there were risks but he was still convinced the surgery was the best route. I suppose it was, given the fact that until the surgery, the doctor felt the cancer was contained on the lung and the cancer unit would have been targeting one area instead of a couple different areas. So, perhaps it was a blessing things ended up the way they did. Time will tell.

Dad also mentioned several people from the community had been in to see him. Not enough to tire him but enough to brighten the day. So many people care about Dad and Mom. I told a visitor at the hospital last Monday that, while he is my Dad, I feel like he belongs to everyone. He is known far and wide and has helped people from all walks of life. Dad is someone that nobody expected to age or get sick. I know that isn't reasonable but Dad never showed the public when he wasn't feeling well. He just kept going. He is who he has always been; a mover and a shaker. Forty-nine years-ago they moved to Sharbot Lake as newlyweds and immediately began becoming a part of the community. They joined the United Church and Dad has been a member of the Board of Stewards and an Elder since before I was born. He belonged to the school board, council and county council and all the committees associated with these. He and Mom frequently attended dances and the dinners sponsored by local organizations and were always willing to lend a hand and wasn't afraid to put some muscle into whatever he was asked to do. He would be one of the first people to greet a newcomer to the community and very often he was a pallbearer to people who were leaving the community for the last time. He is strong and dependable and so very wise. I'm not just biased. The visits and best wishes from so many emphasize this fact. I am a very lucky person to be his daughter and I will forever be trying to live according to his example.

## Friday, July 8, 2005

*I* spoke to Cathy, at length, yesterday afternoon. Apparently things aren't quite as rosy as Dad tried to make us believe in his e-mail. I reread that letter so many times and said to Gail that it just didn't sound like Dad. Something didn't sound quite right.

Apparently Dad overdid it on Monday when he got home from the hospital. He's trying so hard to make everyone, himself included, believe everything is normal. He was up fairly early and when he got home to Sharbot Lake he was up and down the stairs and made several trips outside. Early Tuesday morning Dad's stomach became upset. He can't keep anything on his stomach and retches even when there is nothing there. He won't have a nap in the afternoon because he's afraid that he won't sleep at night. But he isn't anyway. Afternoon naps are as foreign to Dad and Mom's way of life as rising early on Saturday mornings are to me! Cathy told him to listen to his body. If it says "nap," then he must nap. He also needs to drink more fluids to ward off dehydration.

Dad is only taking a half a Tylenol to keep his pain under control. Dad has never been one to take medicine and all he ever needed to get rid of a headache was half a Tylenol. Cathy went to Dr. Bell's office to see if he'll give her something stronger than Gravol to settle Dad's stomach. Dr. Bell gave Cathy the same medication, in pill form, Dad had been given through IV in the hospital. It will also make him drowsy and perhaps allow him to get some sleep. Hopefully, Mom will sleep, too.

While Cathy was in with Dr. Bell she asked him if withdrawal from the morphine would cause an upset stomach. The doctor didn't think Dad had been on it long enough to cause that kind of a reaction. Dr. Bell felt Dad's system wasn't used to all the medication it

had been on since the surgery and possibly it was upsetting his system. Cathy also mentioned that Dad hasn't had any sort of a reaction since learning about the cancer. He has been brave and strong
and very matter-of-fact when discussing his condition. Perhaps he
has been keeping so much inside and his stomach is now upset or, as
Mom would describe it as "stomach nerves." I think it is a very valid
point and I'm really glad Cathy mentioned it. Dad has an appointment this afternoon and Mom wants Dad to go into the appointment without her in case there is something he wishes to express or
discuss when it is just the doctor and him.

Cathy also said when one of his visitors, which our family knows
very well, came to see him on Wednesday he dissolved into tears.
Mom said she hadn't seen it coming and their visitor was taken off
guard. I think it could have a lot to do with post operative depression and perhaps a little bit to do with the emotions he's kept bottled up for so long. Maybe it's a good thing for him to be able to
express his emotions although it's very difficult to watch someone
who has always been so strong and always there for others who need
strength and support.

The Cancer Center called and has made an appointment with Dad
for July 21. That's a Thursday and I'm thinking, if I can arrange it,
I'd like to be with them. There's strength in numbers, right?

This is such a difficult time. I want to be with them yet when I am I
don't know what to say or do to help. I was thinking about what I
said regarding Dad being someone who belongs to many people. He
has never been impressed with titles although he has held many in
his lifetime. The three titles which are the most important to him
are those of husband, father and grandfather. Those are the titles he
is the proudest of.

Dad has known many people from all walks of life. He can easily strike a conversation with someone sitting next to him. He has always had an interest in people and the stories they've had to tell. People are interesting. Dad has known people with important jobs but he is quick to remind us that important jobs don't make important people.

Dad feels people are basically good and that given a chance will rise to the occasion. He believes in encouragement and praise. Dad understands that people are human and will make mistakes and poor choices. He also knows there is a small element of people who take pleasure in doing things which cause pain and are not happy unless they are gossiping or putting down an achievement. There are people who delight in making trouble between friends and family. He has taught us to watch-out for these people. They can be closer than we think. He believes in hard work and not expecting others to provide for you. He always said he'd never ask someone else to do something he wouldn't do himself. He believes in being fair and keeping your business inside your own house. He doesn't believe in wearing his good fortune on his nose for everyone to see. He doesn't believe in discussing other people's business. He has always said "they can buy whatever they want as long as they aren't asking me to pay the bill." In other words, it's none of his business. Dad believes there truly is a time for everything and the natural order of life works only because there is a time for everything. He has worked hard and he's had some lucky opportunities but he'd never consider himself better than the next guy. His greatest pleasure is having the family around for any possible reason and knowing, without exception, that we want to be together. He takes the greatest kick out of surprising us. It pleases him beyond words to know that Cathy, Gail and I are close friends and stay in frequent contact. He and Mom are proud of the fact that our entire family can consider each other to be friends, supporters, advisors, critics and confidantes. That's our way. Gail said during Dad's surgery that Dad may be the one on the table but Dr Reid was going to have to cut through all our hearts to get to Dad's lung.

Every Christmas when we ask him what he'd like his answer is the same every year, "our family's health, being together and Mom's Christmas dinner." When I was a kid I would be so unimpressed. How would I wrap-up that gift? As an adult, I understand what he meant, and now, that's all I want for any day of the year; our health, our family and Mom's Christmas dinner.

All the strength he has shown us, and other people, will now be required to fight this horrid disease. All the lessons he has taught us by word and by example will guide us through this time of fear and uncertainty.

I've had a number of people ask me about Dad. Sometimes it's really easy to say "He's doing fine. Thanks for asking." Other times it's far from being easy.

## July 11, 2005

*It's* been record heat all week and it's continued through the weekend. Perfect cottage weather! Ron and I stained the deck and shutters on Saturday and Sunday. We worked hard but enjoyed the time together. Greg spent the weekend at our friends' cottage on Georgian Bay. Brandon had his friend Nigel spend the night so it felt like Ron and I had the weekend for us. I looked forward to having everyone home under the same roof at the end of the weekend.

I had a lengthy conversation with Cathy on Friday evening. She called to fill us in on Dad's appointment and how he was feeling.

The anti-nausea medication seemed to be helping. Mom and Dad had a good sleep and Dad was eating and drinking everything in sight. He especially seemed to like food that was salty which is good to increase his blood pressure and make him thirsty. Cathy had checked this and it was improving. Cathy said he sounded stronger and looked better although he was still pale. Steve and Cathy dropped in to Mom and Dad's a few times during the day to see how they were doing. His appointment at Dr. Bell's, which included Mom because that was what Dad wanted, seemed to go well. Dr. Bell spent over a half hour with Mom and Dad and the nature of the visit seemed almost a counselling session. The doctor asked Dad if he felt he had to protect our feelings and if he could be honest expressing his feelings with Mom and the rest of us. Dad felt he not only could, but, he had been. The three of them talked about a range of things pertaining to Dad's cancer and Mom and Dad felt very good when they left the office.

I asked Cathy if she felt I should plan on coming down next weekend and she thought it would be better to wait until he was feeling better. She also didn't think Dad would want me to come down for the appointment at the Cancer Center. Cathy is doing what she thinks is best and I thanked her. I also told her I felt like the door to Mom and Dad had temporarily closed. I don't want to call in case they are having a chance to rest. Dad answers his e-mail sporadically and I'm not there to visit. My only contact is through Cathy. I told Cathy that she had the credentials which allowed her access to doctor appointments and to Dad. Cathy is really being so good and patient and understanding. It's just the challenge of having a parent who is unwell and I live at a distance. We've always been so close and whenever I feel like chatting to them I pick up the phone. Now, I think about whether this would be a good time to call or not.

Gail also called me on Friday evening. She and Cathy had talked earlier in the day and they had decided, to save Cathy from repeating herself, that Gail would call Cathy to get the news about Dad's appointment and then Gail would pass the information along to me. We talked for well over an hour. I filled her in on my feelings and we discovered we were each feeling the same way. We feel cut off from Mom and Dad. We decided that Cathy would keep us informed and giving Mom and Dad a little space to help Dad recover is the right thing. But, it will be hard.

Mom and Dad called us on Saturday morning just as we were getting ready to start the deck. It was wonderful to hear them both sounding so much better. They each spoke to both Ron and I. They are hoping to be able to spend some time at the cottage this summer and I can't wait to get them here so we can fuss over them a little. Dad can't drive for a month but Steve and Cathy would bring them here or we'd go and pick them up from Sharbot Lake. The logistics really isn't too hard to figure out. I told them I'd call on our regular Sunday morning routine but Dad said they'd call us in case he was resting and he didn't want to miss the call. I felt much better about getting our day started after talking to them.

Mom called again on Sunday sounding even more rested. I didn't get a chance to talk to Dad because someone dropped by to visit him just as they called. Mom said he was doing much better and he would likely write to me on Monday with the computer. I can't wait to hear from him.

On Saturday evening Ron and I were just relaxing outside after finishing up the first coat on the deck when Ron's brother and sister-in-law, Steve and Dawn, dropped by for a visit. Their daughter, Melody and a friend had come by earlier by seadoo. Steve and Dawn hadn't been there long when another friend dropped by. He stayed for about a half hour and had a little visit with Steve whom he knows, too. It was really nice to have people find their way to our door and have a visit. We really enjoy that aspect of cottage life. Everyone is so casual and relaxed and it is easy to welcome friends and family into our summertime retreat.

On Sunday Ron brought his father, Allie, out to our cottage for dinner. He had had a cataract removed on Thursday and we didn't want him to drive himself. Ron did a good job at the grilling the pork loin chops.

Greg came home around 8pm. Ron took Nigel home at 9pm. It was a full weekend.

I told Gail and Ron the cottage was someplace I can go and, while I don't forget about Dad's illness, I can put it in second place and not be so worried. The cottage is my haven and my spot of peace and happiness. I hated to leave that wonderful spot this morning to come back to work. The temperature is supposed to reach well past the 30 C degree mark so the cottage is definitely the place to be. The weekend had been a scorcher but we didn't mind the heat because of the breeze from the lake and the shade the maples provided. We didn't even get burned while staining the deck. I left the boys there this morning when I went to work. They want to come into town at lunchtime for a couple of hours and then return with Ron when he is finished at the store. I have council tonight so I might just stay at our house until my meeting. We'll see how hot I get. I may need a swim in the lake before tonight's meeting.

## Wednesday, July 13, 2005

*I've* heard from Dad everyday this week and each day his e-mail sounds a little more like "Dad". They've had a lot of company which is very kind and thoughtful for people to take the time from their day to visit but visiting can also be tiring. He's been taking a little nap in the afternoons to recover and recoup his strength.

Cathy and the kids stopped to visit Mom and Dad for a few minutes. Brad was going to cut the grass behind Mom and Dad's and Lindsay was on her way to work. It's nice they live so close. They've been able to have little visits all their lives and that has been great for Mom and Dad, too.

My boys stay close by phoning Mom and Dad often. Greg and Dad have had many conversations regarding his math and applying himself. He and Grandpa have discussed an unfair teacher, a subject he needs extra help in and putting his "shoulder to the wheel" and getting the job done with or without the teacher's help. Greg took his math book down to Arden in June to show Grandpa his progress. Grandpa asks about his class every Sunday on the phone and we report test results as we get them. Last night Greg received his report card in the mail. He opened the card in the privacy of the cottage and emerged a few minutes later with his face beaming but also just a little afraid to believe what he was seeing. He got all his credits, including his math credit. Greg's average had improved from the end of the third term to a 57. The class average in math had dropped from a 55 to a 53. He earned every one of those 57 marks. He went to a tutor twice a week. He studied. He worked hard. And now, he received his reward! After the shock wore off the first thing he said was, "Can I call Grandpa and Grandma? I want to tell them I passed my math class." He was so proud when he told Mom and Dad and they were thrilled for him and proud of him. It's really nice to see someone work really hard for something and get what they were striving for. I was afraid he'd not get the credit and then say, "What good did going to a tutor do for me?" I was afraid it would knock his confidence. This passing mark tells him that he can do anything if he wants it badly enough and is prepared to work for it. Ron and I are so thrilled for him. Every time I look at him I can see the relief in his face!

## Friday, July 15, 2005

*We're* still experiencing a heat wave.

Dad's fine. His e-mail yesterday indicated they had been to the farm with Cathy and Bradley in the afternoon. Mom and Dad supervised while Cathy and Brad cut the grass and trimmed around the property.

I'm feeling quite antsy or unsettled today. I'm trying to think positive but last night I was reading, quite by accident, an article in last Augusts' Chatelaine magazine about cancer and cancer treatments. The article mentioned many side effects I wasn't aware of. I knew the possibility of hair loss and upset stomach but I was unaware that he could swell which could distort his face features. His skin may become extremely thin or very dry and scaly. Any smell or thought of food may be uninviting. There are just so many things which maybe a side effect. The changes will be dramatic for me because I won't be there to see him changing on a daily basis.

I'm also working very hard at learning how to relax and how to savor the moment. I have always been someone who makes plans.

I've always said the best part of a vacation is the planning and the looking forward to it. Now, I don't feel as though I can make plans too far into the future and because of that I am feeling a bit boxed in. I'm trying to learn to enjoy the day and to find pleasure and joy in each day. It's harder some days to be positive and recognize joy and good fortune. I try to think happy thoughts but I have to remember everything can change in an instant. A phone call can come at any moment and change our world forever. Look at the call I received from Gail in April regarding Dad. I was expecting a call because she had just finished her final university exam. Instead, the phone rang and I found out our dad had lung cancer and things didn't look good. I keep looking at our boys and wondering what life will hold for them? What will they remember about us? I look at Ron and think how blessed I was to have found him. Would I be able to cope if Ron was diagnosed as having a serious illness? He is so full of energy. So many people depend on him. He is stable and loving and so very thoughtful. Right now, for this very moment, we are healthy and happy and together. Trying to change my way of looking at the world makes me sad when I realize how temporary our lives really are. I feel like the world has changed and it forgot to ask me if I wanted it to.

I feel very close to tears today. I can't figure out why. Dad is recuperating and seems to be gaining back his strength. There is even some talk that the family may come up to the cottage next weekend depending on how Dad's consultation goes at the Cancer Center on Thursday. The boys are happy and healthy. Greg got his math credit. Friends and family will be around on the weekend. I really haven't any reason to feel so close to tears but I just do. Dad may be the one with the cancer growing inside him but we are all living with cancer and there are a lot of emotions connected with the disease. Colleagues have been a real help. They don't ask about Dad every time I see them but I feel their concern for me. Quiet support is exactly what I need and the people who provide it are many. They may never know how much I have appreciated knowing they are behind me.

## Monday, July 18, 2005

*We* had a nice weekend. A lot of the time was devoted to Greg's roller hockey windup in North Bay Saturday afternoon and Sunday afternoon. They played three games, won the first two and lost the last one. Greg is glad it is over with and wasn't too upset by their loss. In between games we got a lot of work done. Ron made my coffee Saturday and Sunday morning as per usual but it seems to taste so much better at the cottage.

On Friday night we finished painting the window casings at the end of the cottage and made an attempt to paint the front window-shutters. Boy! That window is high off the ground! Ron held the ladder and I volunteered to go up to paint. I won't be so quick to volunteer again! Ron also painted the cedar shakes on the bunkhouse peak. They had been painted white a year ago but needed a little touching up. Some summer neighbors dropped by in their boat for a short visit. Having people drop in off the water is one of the things I really love about the cottage.

After Ron and Greg left Saturday afternoon I worked on laundry, mopped the kitchen floor, put up the last curtain rod and hung the topper, I tidied the boys' room, got groceries, stopped at the LCBO and purchased an outside dining set for the deck. The round, tan-color table seems to fit like it was made for the spot. We ate our first dinner on it when the guys got home from North Bay. I weeded the garden and did some dishes. Brandon and I also went for a few swims. I used my floatie chair for the first time this summer. Brandon tethered me to the dock so I wouldn't float away!

Saturday evening our close friends Curt, Linda and the kids came by for a drink to celebrate the start of their vacation. The weather on Saturday was very hot, continued heat from the start of July and the humidity was at its highest. We chatted and laughed and they stayed until almost midnight. Linda has been privy to my thoughts, concerns and fears regarding Dad via our frequent e-mails. For the evening we didn't discuss Dad's illness and I put on a happy face. Inside, though, I really wasn't in the mood to chat. I was just quietly enjoying their company.

On Sunday I spoke to all my family. We called Dad and Mom at noon which is our usual Sunday routine. Gail had arrived there on Saturday so I had a chance to speak briefly to her. Gail's on holidays and has been out of touch since last Sunday. Dad sounded stronger but tires easily and only stayed on the phone for a few minutes. Mom said things were going well and they were starting to get a bit of sleep at night. For all the brave words I don't believe everything is quite as wonderful as they are trying to make me believe. I've known them too long to not be able to read the unspoken signs.

Allie came for Sunday dinner. He sat chatting about people and happenings from the past and current events until almost 8pm. After Allie left Ron suggested we call Cathy and Steve to see how things are. The days are running together for Cathy. They pop in to see Mom and Dad once a day, more if needed. Dad hasn't been sleeping well and by extension neither has Mom. He has started on the tonic again which may help with his appetite. Cathy says Dad has lost weight. If she has noticed it and she is seeing him every day it must be a substantial weight loss. She says his spirits are good but he seems to have waves of sleepiness and nausea and has to lay down frequently. She didn't feel that he would be strong enough to come to the cottage on the weekend. From everything she said I agreed although deep down I realized I had been hoping they'd be able to visit, more than I knew.

Later, I called Gail after she arrived back at home in Kingston. She said Dad has lost weight, about ten to fifteen pounds. She said Dr Reid had told him he would drop weight while he was healing. He doesn't seem to have a sweet tooth any more but craves salt. He also enjoys a half a beer twice a day. There are calories in the beer and Gail found a can of cashews which are good for him, full of protein and calories and he seemed to like those. Gail also brought a case of a canned meal-supplement made for people who aren't eating. He found the drink too rich straight from the can so Gail cut it down by half with milk and then cut it down some more. She felt he drank it just to amuse her. He isn't drinking nearly as much fluids as Gail and Cathy both would like him to. Gail said he occupies three spaces in the den; the high back sofa chair, the couch and the floor. He needs to sit up and likes the support of the sofa chair, when he needs to lay down he heads to the couch and sometimes he gets unto the floor which seems to feel good on his back. I mentioned we were talking about going down on the weekend since it was obvious he couldn't travel. Gail hesitated and then chose her words very carefully. She felt that having everyone there would be too much for him. He would try to stay up to visit and having that many people would mean someone would be sitting in all his spaces and he wouldn't ask anyone to get up and move. Bed time is early and the boys might not want to go to bed at 9pm and Dad or Mom would stay up until everyone went to bed. I see her point. The confusion alone would be tiring. Perhaps I should consider going down myself for this visit.

I was so upset after talking to both Cathy and Gail that my evening just started to crumble. Brandon has a friend staying over for a couple of nights so I didn't want them to find me in a puddle of tears. On the outside I was keeping it together but as soon as I got into bed I couldn't keep the tears back any longer. Ron held me and let me cry and then he listened as I explained that there hadn't been a day since the end of April that I hadn't cried. Most times I manage to have my moments when I am alone and then appear fine when Ron and the kids are around. Ron knows better but he lets me continue my charade. I told him there is a slow realization that nothing will ever be the same again. Dad's cancer will always be with us. The carefree times we've enjoyed up until now are only a memory. Yes, we've been blessed. This is the only serious illness we have ever had to deal with. Knowing that doesn't make this any easier. I also realized that everything Ron and I have been doing at the cottage this year was to show Dad. He has always had an interest in what the family is up to and he has always enjoyed helping us by doing whatever he can. Last year, when the Clark family came north to our cottage, Dad was first man on the roof of the shed getting things ready to replace it with a steel roof. He had made a shopping list for Ron the autumn before and Ron had all the materials ready for the workbee. Now, there is doubt that he will be strong enough to even visit this summer. What I wouldn't give to see him get out of the car and walk down the path to the cottage!

I've also become so over protective with Ron and the boys. I was always over protective but I'm fanatical now. I worry about everything. I worry about the bears getting into the bunkhouse, about the chipmunks chewing the electrical wires, about the boys hitting their heads on something as they fool around in the lake. I worry they may get hurt playing roller hockey or ice hockey. I worry they'll be hit by a car on their bikes. I worry about Ron. He's almost fifty-one and his Dad has a heart problem and his Mom died from a heart attack and her heart had always been strong. I worry whenever he sleeps too much or he looks too tired. I worry he is working too hard. I worry he's on the road too much. I worry if I haven't heard from him. I worry about everything. The boys are starting to chafe with all my worries and rules and restrictions. Ron comes to their rescue without taking sides. He helps ease the restrictions and seems to understand that I need to protect my loved ones from the things I can control because I haven't any control over Dad's illness. I even worry that I may be losing my own sanity and my constant worrying will push the boys away.

I'm afraid I just can't focus on anything today except Dad and our family. I've wiped tears away all morning and hope my eyes aren't red when someone comes into the office to see me. I would feel so silly if they caught me in tears and yet I can't seem to get straightened around. I'm trying to work but everything I do I find myself having to do three times to get it right. I shouldn't even be here in this state. I should be out at the cottage but Patty is on vacation and Raina is here until 2pm so I'm the only one left at the counter after she leaves. I would love to be at the cottage sitting under one of the maple trees and watching the boys. I hate being away from the cottage. We have made it into such a happy place with its colourful fabrics and whimsical extras we have sprinkled around the property. Last week I attached a resin "face" to a tree. It is subtle and blends in with the bark but definitely stands out when we look for it. There are several shades of blue and shots of red and yellow all around the property. The flower pots have the same colors in them which add to the festive atmosphere. I'd just like to sit outside in a lounge chair and retreat into my thoughts. I realize the value of every minute of a day but I can't wait to get back to the cottage this evening to be with my family and in my "happy" surroundings.

Ron knows how difficult my weekend was and he has checked in on me a couple of times today to see "how things were going." I can't imagine going through this without him at my side. His mother went so suddenly and we didn't have any time to even think about what it will be like without her. We didn't have time to get over the shock. And, most important, we didn't watch her suffer because she didn't. She was comfortable and the night before she died she was visiting with Ron's youngest brother in her hospital room. She died peacefully and the quickness of her death was a blessing for her as well as those of us who loved her. The difficult part was later; when reality set in. It was when she wasn't sitting in her rocking chair watching for us to come in for a visit or when I set two extra places at the dinner table instead of one. I hope I was some comfort to Ron during that horrible time. I tried to help our boys deal with life's reality in a way they could understand. I was trying to cope with the loss myself.

I feel like I'm drowning. I can't breath; my throat hurts from gasping for air and yet, to the world around me, I'm calm and in control. They don't understand how a song on the radio can trigger my tears or how seeing something as benign as a water pump can cause a flood of memories. Dad is a licensed plumber and when we were younger he had a plumbing business he ran on the weekends and in the evenings. He installed bathrooms, drained pumps in the fall and hooked up the pumps again in the spring time. I watched him tear apart a pump so many times to replace ball bearings or a motor part. I grew up learning to ask people if the pump needed to be reset, "Did you push the button?" Countless widows, who would be on the other end of the phone in a panic looking for Dad because their pump wouldn't stop running, were told by my Mom or my sisters or I to turn off the switch so the motor wouldn't over heat. I am a plumber's daughter. I know what it means to prime a pump. I know that air gets into the waterlines. We spent hours with Dad on the weekend at a cottage when he was installing a bathroom or servicing a pump before the summer season. So now, when I see a pump, there are many happy memories attached. It isn't just a pump; it is an extension of my dad. People don't understand how I can be fine one minute and dissolve into tears a second later. Dad is a man of the world. Everything from shrimp to Red Skeleton-reruns reminds me of Dad and our life together. Mom put it best when she said there was a hole in all our hearts that can't be fixed and we just have to learn to live with that hole. Things will never be the same and part of me still can't believe we have to accept these changes.

I know I've thought this repeatedly but how did we get to this place when four months ago we were in Panama enjoying our time together? Poor health was the furthest thing from all our minds. A serious illness never even crossed our minds. Our parents stopped being "our parents" years ago. What they became, instead, are our dear friends. They are people whose company we enjoy and look forward to spending time with. We have common interests and our likes are similar. They listen, debate and kid around. They're honest and compassionate and will confide in us, too. They are our travel companions, our fiercest supporters, our advisors, our comforters and our children's most loyal friends and devoted grandparents. Every stage of our children's life has been a cause for celebration. They keep our feet on the ground by reminding us what is important and how we did the same things when we were kids. They've attended hockey games and skating carnivals, they've sat through piano concerts and ball games. They were with the children the day they were each born and seldom missed a birthday. They've taken the kids camping and to the zoo and were with them on their first plane ride. Grandma has pulled more baby teeth than any of the parents. They've attended graduations and given pep talks on the merits of studying and working hard. They've watched young adults head off to the prom. They have been involved grandparents in everyway. Not one of the four grandchildren feel left out or neglected. Each one is special and each ones knows it. When our children have a success the first people they have to call is Grandpa and Grandma. They know that whatever they do their grandparents are interested and supportive. Grandma even learned to like hockey just so she'd be able to talk "hockey" when the boys came to visit. Mom and Dad have become so much more than parents. The bonds which tie us are unique and special. All of us have felt the love and warmth and pride they feel for us and because they believe in us so strongly we believe in ourselves and strive to always reach higher. So, watching a parent battle a serious illness is difficult but watching a parent, who is also a close friend, becomes unbearable.

People say that children are too young to remember far off destinations. Our children not only remember but join in the "remember when we were in…." conversations which always seem to emerge during our times together. Our trips haven't just lasted the week we were away but are relived again and again through pictures and conversation. The truly amazing thing about our group is the background may change but we are always gathered together laughing and sharing. Always the focus stays the same, *our family.*

Mom and Dad just celebrated their forty-ninth wedding anniversary. Under normal circumstances we would already be making plans for their fiftieth celebration. We would take great pleasure in planning something for our family and a little something for the community. The event would be filled with happy memories and plans for many more. Now, none of us dare think so far into the future. Any celebration we will have will be poignant and filled with future uncertainty. How did this happen? Why can't I wake up from this nightmare? Why can't someone hear me as I cry in my sleep and realize I'm dreaming a terrible dream? Why won't someone wake me up and tell me it is all a dream? It feels so real. I just have to let the dream unfold until morning comes and I awaken. Then my heart will stop pounding and my tears will finally dry. Then my worlds will be right again and we can start to make plans to be together. I know I'll remember this dream when I awaken. This dream won't be lost in the dawn. I will remember and I will know how lucky we are to have our health and each other.

## Tuesday, July 19, 2005

*The* month of July is quickly disappearing. I feel somewhat more settled today then I did yesterday.

I arrived back at the cottage to find Ron had brought me something. Last Sunday I had wanted a lemon pie for dinner. I found a nice, delicious one at the grocery store and decided to bring it home. When I cut into it at dinner I discovered it wasn't lemon, after all, but key lime. I guess I didn't look very hard. Ron had been to North Bay yesterday and saw a lemon pie and he brought it home for me. He is so thoughtful. I had a piece after my swim and it was every bit as good as it looked.

Tracy and Mike McCron and their friend, Sandra and Wayne Murray, came by boat for a visit in the evening. It was nice to sit around and laugh. One of the things I love about the cottage is how casual it is and how easy to entertain. People drop by in the boat more often then by car but nobody fusses and after having a little visit they head out. Having a cottage where nobody comes would be so sad.

A friend's daughter is to be married in August in Ottawa. Ron and I were talking about it last night. I mentioned that he might want to get a new sports jacket and shirt since the summer has been so hot I know he'll swelter in his suit. I still have to find something for me to wear but, truthfully, as much as I was looking forward to this wedding I can't seem to get excited about it at all. However, we will be able to spend time with Mom and Dad which makes it a bit easier. I love Ottawa in the summertime but this year I can't seem to enjoy things the way I normally would.

It would be easy to confuse me with someone who has already lost her father but I think I'm still coming to terms with our new reality and mourning the end of our existing way of life. I am finding joy in my day which is a big accomplishment on some days. I always love to see the loons in the bay and watch the little family of ducks when the mother takes them out for an evening swim. I find pure joy in listening to our boys laugh and giggle as they play in the water and Ron is a great source of joy. Ron doesn't leave my side unless he has to take one of the boys somewhere. That's another thing I love about the cottage. We have time to be a couple. If the weather holds today we have decided we'd like to go for a kayak ride after dinner.

Our boys are growing so tall and becoming such lovely young men. They still drive me nuts when they drop wet towels and clothes and mess up a room as fast as I can clean it but, they are thoughtful and sensitive and I believe they will become very caring men. They are each so different from one another yet each offers the family something extremely precious. I am so proud of those two. Everyone has said what nice, polite young men they are. I hope they know, even when I'm being hard on them, how much they mean to me and how my life has been blessed by their arrival into it.

I'm just emotionally "on hold" until I see how Dad makes out with his radiation and chemotherapy. The only emotions which seem alive and well are fear, love, protectiveness and profound sadness. I seem to be reviewing the past, fearing the future and at the same time I'm living the present one minute at a time. Perhaps, after Dad's treatments have finished I will find a spark again. Dad won't like this if he were to know how I'm feeling. He would not want to be the reason I am feeling so "down". Dad has made a life by taking it by the horns and "going for it". We all have set backs and disappointments but life is for living. I can just hear him saying that. Hopefully I can work through this stage of "coming to terms". Hopefully, I don't drive myself and everyone around me crazy before I do! Hopefully, I can get this flood of emotion under control before I travel to see them this weekend. I'm the eldest daughter. I have to gain some composure and not look like a sobbing fool when I'm there. I've always been so sentimental and emotional. A family friend told me once that the two of us were similar; we both had our tear ducts attached to our bladders!

I had better get busy with my paying job. There is much to accomplish before I leave on vacation in nine days. The sound of the word "vacation" sounds so soothing and peaceful. The weekends go by quickly. Having seven days in a row to enjoy the cottage and the people I care about so much will be like a brief visit to Heaven. This is part of the reason I want to go to Sharbot Lake this weekend. I need to see Dad because when I saw him last he hadn't been up for a walk and was still hooked up to tubes, etc. in the hospital. I need to see him up and about even though he isn't back to how he was before the surgery. I have to see him! I need to be with Mom and

Dad. Then, once I have been there I can relax a bit and enjoy our vacation without travelling. Travelling is tiring; especially if you aren't sleeping well to begin with.

This journal has been a great way for me to get my thoughts out and examine them as they develop. I've said it before but this illness is a learning experience for all of us and finding a way to take positive lessons from it is the purpose of life. I've no doubt that my perspective on life will change dramatically the further down this road we travel. Everyone's view of life changes with maturity and experience. So, it will be interesting to look back upon these words, even in six months, and see how far I have come as well as the changes our family will go through.

## Wednesday, July 20, 2005

---

Subject: Re:Hi!
Date:     2005 Jul 20 11:39
From:   Harold Clark
To:      Susan Arnold

Hi, Susan

Yes, we spend a lot of time out on the hill watching the boats on the lake. It helps with the fresh air but it's nice to get back inside to cool off every little while. We are still experiencing restless nights and poor appetite which explains the listless and tired feeling, however, it will gradually get better.

Mom is busy making cookies and doing things in the house besides looking after me. It was cooler last night than usual; about 18 when we got up this morning but it is suppose to go back up to 29 again today.

**Nothing else of news here so will run along.**

**Take care, have a good day, say Hi to all and we will talk to you later.**

**Love Mom and Dad**

I received a lengthy e-mail from Gail yesterday afternoon. She and Cathy have been so good about staying in touch with me. They understand how difficult it is when they are close so it must be harder when I'm at a distance. Cathy explains medical facts and jargon and Gail tells me exactly what she sees and shows me the big picture.

Gail said Dad's colour was getting better. He didn't feel as winded when he goes for his little walks around the property. His appetite is starting to pick up but it's not stellar yet. She indicated healing takes a lot of calories and since he isn't feeling much like eating he is just getting the calories he needs and no more. Once his healing is complete he should start to put on some weight. She feels he is on the mend although it is going to take some time and we may just be in the calm before the storm. His appointment at the cancer center is tomorrow so they will fill him in on when, where and how.

We have also decided I am going to have a solo flight to Sharbot Lake this weekend. I need to see them both and spend time with them. The unsettling part of that statement is I really don't want to go in these circumstances. I feel very inadequate and not sure what to say or do. Both Cathy and Gail intimidate me with how easily they know what to do to provide comfort. I admire them for their poise and their confidence. I feel like I just fumble along doing what I'm told to do or what I've seen done before. Cathy is a trained nurse and Gail has taken courses about death and dying at university. I've never had an interest in such things. Now I wish I had.

I'd rather not talk about Dad's cancer but Mom and Dad aren't people who deny the facts. They don't dwell on it, but I won't be able to avoid it, either. The next thing is Dad's weight loss. It will be a shock seeing him so much thinner then he was even in the hospital.

And the third thing, the most difficult thing, will be trying to control my own emotions for the entire weekend. I can't let them see me in the state I've been in for the past week. Obviously, Cathy will be stopping-in from time to time but there will also be a fair amount of one-on-one time with Mom and Dad. So, when Cathy is around I will have a buffer but the rest of the time I will be on my own without anyone there to run interference for me.

Gail has mentioned Dad grazes a lot when something tastes good to him. Last week it was cashews. He seems to have lost his sweet tooth and prefers something salty. Ron is going to pick up some cashews for me at the bulk store tomorrow so I can take them down with me on Friday. So, I'm going to pop into a health food store and pick up a container of protein powder. Mom can make him a shake and can add whatever he might like to augment the flavor. I often add a banana or strawberries or, if his sweet tooth returns, he can add chocolate syrup. He can mix it with milk or juice or Mom can add it to yogurt and muffins. Anything we can do to get the protein into him will be a benefit. I'm going to throw in a bag of mini-carrots and grape tomatoes to snack on. Obviously, empty calories won't help him but the salt helps raise his blood pressure, the protein helps with his muscle and the vitamins and minerals from the vegetables will also help in many areas. Mom has gotten him back taking a tonic which will build up his immune system and fight the cancer cells. I must check to see if they will need more before I come down.

Dad sent an e-mail yesterday, too. His e-mails are so short and bland. There doesn't seem to be any interest or colour in them. He mentions they've had company but doesn't mention who visited. He doesn't answer questions I've asked and rarely comments about things I'm telling him. I'm trying to keep my e-mails light and filled with our activities but I get the feeling he is replying with a duty e-mail and has no interest in what I actually write.

I have absolutely no interest in my work or a desire to even be here. I'd rather spend my time with my husband, my boys and people I care about. Perhaps I'm just more than ready for my vacation. Perhaps I just see my work as an interruption in my life. When I've reached the end of my life what regrets will I have? Will I regret not keeping my filing up to date? I rather doubt it! The boys are growing so fast. Greg will turn fifteen in September and Brandon is twelve. Summers with them will soon be only small amounts of time away from jobs. Already they are making plans which don't include their Dad and me. I should be there at the lake having fun with them instead of lecturing them about messy rooms and extra laundry. I know they are teenagers. Teenagers aren't known for their neatness. They aren't any different from others. In fact, they're probably much better behaved then many. Yet, I seem to get my buttons pushed and the anger inside me because of Dad, because of the job, because of my own hormonal changes all swirl together and erupt when all of us least expect it. Its sudden arrival even surprises me. What starts out as a small thing escalates so quickly I can't believe it is me talking. I worry about that, too.

I just received an e-mail from Cathy. She sounds more stressed and concerned then normal. I had sent her a message earlier telling her I was planning to come to Sharbot Lake on Friday and she responded by saying she thought that was a great idea. She said there is some-thing going on with Dad and she can't put her finger on it. He's lost 23 pounds since the end of May. Cathy said she asked him directly if Thursday's appointment at the Cancer Center will ease his mind about what will happen once he starts his treatments. He didn't answer her and she is afraid he may have given up. She said she asked Mom if she wanted to come to South River and Mom didn't think Dad was up to the drive yet. Cathy then wondered if Mom would like me to come down and even stay at Cathy's place so I don't interrupt their routine too much. Mom said that would be great and Cathy added, again, "just come, Sue". Cathy is dreading tomorrow's appointment yet she wants it to be over with, too.

I felt much better after receiving Gail's e-mail on Tuesday but Cathy's e-mail puts me right back to wondering what is going on. I knew by the tone of his e-mails Monday and Tuesday he wasn't having a good day and Cathy seems to support that idea. I think, in light of this e-mail I should leave South River on Friday as soon as I can. The timing is just all wrong. Normally we'd have staff here all the time and I wouldn't feel bad leaving but Raina has booked Fri-day off for vacation and so did Martin. That only leaves Patty and me. Once September arrives I can head out whenever but summer is hard with everyone trying to get in some vacation time.

I'm starting to feel very tired. My brain never seems to rest. If I'm not thinking about Dad and his cancer I'm thinking about things I need to do here in case I leave suddenly and I'm thinking of things I need to do at the house to make sure we have clothes and groceries. I'm constantly interpreting e-mails and listening for what isn't being said on the telephone. If I'm tired then Cathy must be exhausted. She has been tending to her family, driving Dad and Mom to appointments in Kingston and checking in on them when they are at home. I wish I could be close by to help lighten the load. The mental stress isn't going to go away but the physical stress could be eased and just having someone else to drop in instead of having it all on her shoulders would help her tremendously. I worry about her. I worry about Mom, too. She lives with this nightmare every single day. For her, there is no escape; no chance to allow her emotions to be the priority.

Dad's e-mail has arrived and once again, while it is great to see his name pop up on my screen, there is definitely something missing from his letters. Today I told him I'd received a note from a former teacher. I mentioned we were looking for the best place to put the central vacuum and I mentioned the hurricane heading towards Texas. I asked if they had heard from my uncle in Houston. I asked if they were keeping a guestbook for their visitors and mentioned the appointment tomorrow. He responded with the weather report, Mom's activities, his poor appetite and restless nights and then said to say Hi to all. That was it; short and sweet and so different from his normal e-mail. I really feel he is e-mailing me, not because he wants to, but because he wants to keep me off his back. He knows if I don't hear from him in a couple of days I will be on the phone asking "why". That's not something I've started recently. I've done that for over three years. I'm thinking it could be a delayed post operative depression since it has only been three weeks this past Monday since the surgery. Or, perhaps, it is the reaction he hasn't had to the whole thing, the cancer, the surgery and the enormity of it all which has finally caught up to him. He was so strong and so calm and hardly faltered. Only if we broke down did he miss a step but he was quick to recover. Whatever his private thoughts were, I can't say, but he sure didn't show us any downside. That can't go on forever. He is only human; as much as we hate to admit it.

Focusing on something other than my own emotions and knowing my family needs me has helped shift my thought process from emotional to practical.

I just called Cathy and she filled me in on much of what she had said or alluded to in her e-mail. She said Dad told her he really wasn't interested in opening his e-mail but he knows I'm e-mailing and he really wishes I wouldn't because he doesn't feel like writing a letter every day. Cathy told him I'm at a distance and I worry if I don't hear anything. A little note every couple of days would help ease my concern and would give him something to do. Cathy really thinks the appointment tomorrow will either put his mind at rest about what is going to happen or it is going to have no effect at all which could mean he has given up. She remembers our Grandma Clark, Dad's mother, could drop twenty pounds when she was worried over something and Dad is quite similar in many ways. He really gets upset when Gail or I discuss coming for a weekend which involves taking time-off work. He doesn't want us to take time-off because of him. She also said, since the surgery Dad has said the word "cancer" only once; instead he refers to it as a bump in the road. So, if we are showing up when we normally wouldn't then it just seems to make the cancer all the more real. How could he not want us to spend time with him? He and Mom created this family. He knows that we are tied to each other and the pain of one is the pain of everyone. Besides, Mom can use the support. In a way, it is almost like he is pushing us away.

Cathy said Mom is amazing. She drives the car everywhere and yesterday she took the truck and Dad to the farm and they brought home the two Muskoka-chairs. Cathy also said Mom has said a couple of things to her which seem to say that she is watching him die before her eyes. She seems to have accepted Dad is nearing the end of his life. She doesn't want to go anywhere because she wants to stay near him. The more I hear, the more I understand and the more worried I become.

### Friday, July 22, 2005

*The* news is not good. The appointment at the hospital was exhausting for Dad. The doctor told them the fatigue and the upset stomach was likely cancer-related. He has two lumps which can be seen on his back and side. These may or may not have been there before but because he has lost so much weight we can easily see them now. The doctor feels certain it is cancer. He also said it is a good thing in a bad way. When Dad starts his chemotherapy the lumps will act as indicators to see if it is working.

He will begin chemotherapy on Wednesday providing his strength has been built up and his blood work is OK. The doctor prescribed a steroid which should help settle his stomach and enhance his appetite. There has been no mention of radiation which Gail finds strange. Personally, I don't. They have said this will not cure his cancer but may take away some of the symptoms and make him comfortable. If his health allows them to begin chemotherapy on Wednesday at 10am he will receive a powerful dose and the following week he'll receive a moderate one followed by one week off and then they'll begin the cycle again. Then, after four treatments, I guess they will assess the progress and determine the next step.

Cathy seems relieved I am planning to arrive at Mom and Dad's today. I suddenly seem numb. All the tears I've cried since April couldn't have just dried up so quickly. Perhaps it is shock. When I told Ron about it last night I didn't shed any tears and was actually able to sleep through the night. I find that very strange and hope this emotional novocain keeps my feelings in check until after my visit. I think, deep down, if I focus on what this actually means I will cave. It's best to just skirt over the surface and not delve too deep. I told Gail last night that we have now set the wheels in motion and there is no stopping what will happen next. Our family has taken many wonderful trips together and the memories we made as we visited far off places will last each of us a lifetime. Our family began another journey the end of April and this one will be no less meaningful. Each of us will come away with memories we will always have and we will be on this journey together until we reach whatever destination we're suppose to reach.

## Monday, July 25, 2005

---

Subject: Re: Good Morning!
Date:    2005 July 25—12:09
From:    Harold Clark
To:      Susan Arnold

Hi, Susan

Nice to have you for the visit. Hope I didn't spoil it by lying around. We were also glad to hear your voice when you got home yesterday safe and sound with everything great. We also want to thank you for writing the thank you note. We printed it off and Mom is going over to place it in the paper (as is) right after dinner. All else is as usual here today; had a reasonable night's sleep, good breakfast, went to the dump with Mom after she did her wash this morning and tiding up. Will get off here and try to catch

**up on a few things. Take care. Say Hi to all and have a
good day and evening.**

**Love Mom and Dad**

The weekend was an emotional mix but I'm very proud of myself
because I managed to keep it together and not have any breakdowns
during the time I was with Mom and Dad.

On Friday afternoon I found Dad in an extremely fragile, weakened
condition. He was laying on the couch looking very pale, gaunt and
old. He is so thin there is nothing left to him. He didn't get up or
turn his head when I came in but he did say "Hi, Sue" in that faint
voice we hear when people haven't the strength to speak. I kissed
him and sat in the chair across from him so he could see me but he
soon fell back to sleep. He was content that I had arrived safely. He
was wearing a freshly ironed shirt which reminded me how well
Dad has always worn his clothing and has always taken pride in his
appearance. Cathy popped in soon after my arrival. Dad was visibly
fading and the medication which the doctor had prescribed on
Thursday obviously wasn't taking effect yet. She wanted to wait
until Saturday morning before taking him to emergency because he
did have some of the drug in his system although a lot came back up
Thursday and Friday morning.

By Friday evening he seemed to have a small interest in food and ate
what would normally have been regarded as a pitifully small amount
but, in our eyes, was a huge portion. He had a small piece of Canadian bacon. He had a little scoop of mashed potatoes and a couple
of green beans. He then finished his meal with some plain, red Jell-
O. The next couple of hours would tell the tale and hopefully he
would be able to keep it in his system. He did. He also took a couple

of soda crackers with butter before bed in order to take his anti-nausea pill at bed time which would help him sleep.

As a result he slept well through the night. The first time in days which meant Mom had a better night's rest, too. He ate some breakfast. Not a lot, but more than he'd been getting into him. By lunch time he managed to eat a dish of chicken noodle soup, crackers and a banana.

He seemed to be getting stronger right before our eyes and didn't seem to be sleeping nearly as much. He had several visitors in to see him on Saturday morning and was able to have a short rest in between. His color seemed to be less pale and his eyes were much brighter. On Saturday afternoon we sat out on lounge chairs in the backyard watching the boats on the lake. He was thirsty and had a taste for a beer which I went and got for him. He drank half and then settled down in the family room for a nap which lasted well over an hour.

For dinner he ate a full plate of small amounts. He had some mashed potatoes, Canadian bacon, carrots, corn, salad, a slice of tomato, a piece of cucumber and his Jell-o. In the evening he felt strong enough to take a drive to Cathy and Steve's for a short visit.

Again, on Saturday night he had a reasonably good night's sleep. He also ate an egg and some bacon, some toast, a banana and a coffee for breakfast. This was the biggest meal I had seen him eat and he was sounding much stronger and looked more like Dad. Cathy and Steve dropped in before I left and were surprised at how much better he looked. At this rate, if he continues, I have no doubt they will begin chemotherapy on Wednesday. The downside of the chemotherapy will be he will, once again, experience extreme fatigue and nausea. Just when we take one step forward we seem to get knocked back two steps.

The doctor had also mentioned he would arrange for a palliative nurse to begin visiting Dad to help with any of his side effects and be with Mom and Dad as Dad's illness progresses. The idea of a palliative nurse is extremely upsetting but it is a reality we need to deal with. Dad is not going to get better and everything which is being done now is only to keep him comfortable.

I was emotionally drained by the time I left and my release came in the form of tears all the way home. Brandon seemed to need to be with me and didn't leave Ron or me for two minutes the first couple of hours after my return. Greg asked how Grandpa was and then stayed by himself out in the bunkhouse. This is hard on me but the kids and Ron are dealing with their emotions, too, and I'm trying to be sympathetic to what they need from me. I really want to reassure them that I maybe sad and stressed but I love them dearly and want to create a feeling of a "safe haven" within our walls. As long as we are together we'll be fine. Family is everything; that was how both Ron and I were raised.

Ron BBQ'd steaks and did a great job of it, too. We had a good dinner, just the four of us as Allie didn't feel up to travelling to the cottage for our regular Sunday dinner but we had some laughs and I heard all about their shopping trip to North Bay and their activities while I was away.

Gail called me just after I finished the dishes and I think we may have talked for almost two hours. She is going to Dad and Mom's to stay tonight. I told her, basically, he was much better when I left him on Sunday then when I arrived on Friday.

Mom seems resigned to the inevitable but is coping quite well. She is devoting her day to caring for Dad. She doesn't spend her time dwelling on what the future holds and she seems to be managing. She spends a lot of time touching Dad. They hold hands, she rubs his shoulder, his back, his arm and knee. It is as if she is storing him up for the rest of her life. But, I try not to think like that and just continue on with whatever task is at hand to make life easier and more comfortable for both Mom and Dad.

One of the things they had asked me to do was to write thank you notes to people who had brought gifts. He has received two lovely quilts; one was store bought and one was made for cancer patients by a local group and they wanted Dad to have it. Apparently, Mom and Dad think I'm the wordy one! We finished the notes on Saturday night and I dropped them through the mail chute at the post office to go out in today's mail. They have also asked me to write a thank-you to be placed in the North Frontenac Newspaper to thank everyone for their kind words, visits, calls, cards and prayers during his time in the hospital and since his return home. I wrote that note out this morning and e-mailed it down to them. If it is what he likes he need only print it off and Mom or Cathy can drop it off at the newspaper office. If he'd like some revisions he can indicate what they are and return it to me for the final copy. I haven't heard back from them. I hope they've had another good day and night. He needs as much sleep and food as he can get into him to prepare for Wednesday.

I cried from the moment I woke up this morning until I arrived at the office. I had a brief moment with Patty in my office but otherwise I seem to be in control. The day is going to be long as I have a

Council meeting this evening so I have to conserve my energy to make it last.

I have a hair appointment at 1 pm today which will help give me a positive outlook. A trip to the hairdresser always helps. I noticed on the bathroom scales this morning that I am down two pounds. I'll have to watch that I don't go any lower. I need my strength for myself, my boys and my parents.

Dad e-mailed this afternoon. His e-mail was a little longer so that indicates he is feeling better and strong enough to be at the computer. He liked the thank-you note, as is, and printed it off. Mom was going to drop it off at the paper this afternoon. His e-mail indicated he had had a relatively good rest last night and enjoyed another good breakfast. With that type of progress I'm sure he'll be ready to start chemotherapy on Wednesday. However, I'm learning quickly what I said at the beginning of this; just when things seem good or to be improving they deteriorate. When things get worse they suddenly improve. There are many hills and valleys on this road.

## Tuesday, July 26, 2005

---

**Subject: Re: Hi, Cath**
**Date:**   2005 Jul 26—8:55
**From:**   **Cathy Fox**
**To:**       **Susan Arnold**

Hi, Susan

When I dropped in yesterday, Dad seemed to be better. He was doing a word search! His voice is stronger and his colour is better. He's eating about the same as the weekend, which is good. He said he has one episode nauseas/weakness a day and around noon. He lays down and sleeps for less than an hour and then gets up and eats. His knees are less weak. I just hope it improves over today and he will be able to have the chemo. Sleeping about the same; up and down all night, but less restless.

Steve is going to sit down with Dad and make a list of things needing to get down. We were at Seeley's Bay at Brad's ball game last night until 11 pm. Mom and Dad were looking forward to Gail coming out last night. I have to do groceries today and will pop in like I always do. Once Dad starts chemo, we will have to be careful about infection; people with colds, etc. I'm going to pick up a digital thermometer today at the pharmacy so they're all ready. He will have to take his temperature two times a day; at least that was the protocol when I was working.

I'll e-mail Gail so she can let me know how she thought he was. I'll give you an update before the day's out.

See ya,

Love Cathy

*Mom* and Dad were looking forward to Gail's visit last night. I'll have to investigate time off under the compassionate care leave which is like a maternity leave through Employment Insurance but it is for six weeks and I want to save that until the end of Dad's illness. Gail will, I'm sure, be taking similar time but I'll discuss it with her at some point.

I was somewhat better this morning and only had a few tears while I was getting ready to leave the cottage. I keep looking around and seeing all the things I want Dad to see and I keep imagining all the fun our family was suppose to have here this summer. All the fun we were suppose to have for many summers to come seems to have evaporated, leaving instead, ghosts of what might have been.

I also struggled for the briefest of moments at the Kwik Way. A friend asked me how Dad was doing. He was very kind and thoughtful but it just about did me in. I seem to have developed a protective shell to go out into public and when something penetrates the shell I just about shatter.

Gail just e-mailed to tell me Dad had a bad evening yesterday. He had been good until sometime in the afternoon after Lindsay and Cathy left. She said he had a wave of nauseous. He laid on the couch with a cold cloth on his head and slept until around 9:30PM. Then he got up and ate a piece of toast and some grapes before going up to bed. She said he slept pretty well and was only up once that she heard. He had an emotional moment when Gail came to say good bye and said he didn't want to put all this onto the family. She hugged him and said we're all in this together and not to give up. He said he wouldn't. He told her not to be late for work and to drive carefully and, as always, call when she got there. Gail, like me, cried all the way to Kingston. She called at 8:30am and by then Dad was sitting at the table having breakfast with Mom.

This damn disease! I could just scream! Why should someone's final days, weeks, months or years in this world be a time when they are constantly nauseous or in pain? Death must truly be a welcome relief when it comes. When we are in good health, and we have a bout with the flu bug, we feel terrible and we really don't care about anything expect making the queasy feeling in our stomach go away. We know it is only a temporary situation and can suffer through it. How must it feel to know this is nauseous sensation is going to last the rest of our days?

---

Subject: Re: Good Morning!
Date:    2005 Jul 26—11:58
From:   Harold Clark
To:      Susan Arnold

Hi, Susan

You had a bigger dip in temperatures then we did; the lowest we got down to was 72. We had a good visit with Gail although I was somewhat the same as you found me when you came down last Friday. Just one of those days. We will see how everything goes tomorrow. I hope OK.

It has been like juniper junction around here this morning. A man from the church brought us in some fresh honey. My cousins were in for a visit and I think a former employee is coming this afternoon. We had a reasonable nights sleep and a good breakfast this morning. I hope this continues.

We are getting along fine and will be in touch after tomorrow. No other news so will skip along. Have a good day and we will talk later.

Love Mom and Dad

---

If there is anything good to come out of this horrible event it is how much closer our already close family is drawing ... all twelve of us. For each of us the words "I love you" are more frequently used. Moments of tenderness are not rushed in favor of being somewhere else. The sweetness of having "time" is not lost in the hectic schedules of daily life. My sisters and I, all of us independent beings, need each other and we're not afraid to admit it. Ron and Steve have always felt like family but now they feel like they are blood relatives and are willing to do whatever it takes to help any of us. Rob needs us as he goes through his own painful good bye to his Dad. He understands the closeness our family and recognizes it is special and he takes pictures to help us preserve it. My little family treats each other with a consideration and respect we didn't always have time for. Gail and I have always discussed so many things from soup to nuts but our discussions have reached a new level of understanding. Mom and Dad are witnessing what their love for each other has created. Family is everything and now everything else seems unimportant and lacks urgency. As Gail told Dad this morning it is truly "all for one". There is no mistaking the love, devotion and commitment to each other. It shines through in our every action and our every thought. I can't imagine it ever returning to what we had considered normal. We have journeyed to a new relationship which is preparing for the first break in our earthly family.

Gail asked if I would help word something for the newspaper to announce her graduation from Queen's University. Dad and Mom want her picture and announcement put into the paper even though Gail feels sort of "funny" about being the focus of attention when Dad is sick. I told her it isn't about her. They are very proud of their daughter; a Queen's University graduate! They want a happy family announcement and they want to share it together. I agreed to write something out for her and just now sent her a foolish draft! I wish I was on the other end to see her face when she reads it! I hope it gives her a chuckle!

## Wednesday, July 27, 2005

*The* 27th seems to be taking on a life of its own. One month ago today we were at the hospital for Dad's surgery. Today he is starting chemotherapy. I know he began treatments because Cathy had stepped out of the hospital to call Gail to tell her the chemotherapy would proceed as scheduled. Apparently, he is strong enough to withstand the strongest blast of chemotherapy; I've forgotten which drugs are being used today. When people hear the word "chemotherapy" the usual assumption is one drug is administered to the patient with very severe side effects. In actual fact, chemotherapy is a cocktail of cancer-fighting drugs that are tailored to the patient's individual needs. For this reason the patient must have his blood work done on the day of the treatment. The lab will then prepare the drug combination which is appropriate for the patient on that particular day. Chemotherapy is becoming more refined as research continues. The chemotherapy session today will take about five hours. The first two hours will be spent hydrating Dad with a saline solution. The next hour he will have an anti-nausea drug, as well as an antihistamine, administered intravenously. Then they will begin the actual cancer drugs. He should be finished around 4:30 this afternoon or probably closer to five o'clock. The treatment began at 11:30 this morning although he had to be at the lab by eight thirty in the morning for his blood work to be done.

They also cleared up the uncertainty regarding radiation. The doctors decided, since they found the cancer to be more extensive, they would begin with the chemotherapy which would, in effect, spread a net throughout his body and kill any undetected cancer cells and contain what is there. Then, after the chemo is complete, radiation will be done to target the large tumor to reduce its size and help control his symptoms which should improve his quality of life. I feel somewhat better about having that explained. It sounded so bleak after last week's appointment. Perhaps we can buy some precious time when we aren't sitting around praising him when he manages to keep down a slice of bread. Dad has always enjoyed his food and these tiny portions and lack of interest in food is so difficult. Perhaps we can buy some time when Dad can laugh and be with the family. Above all else, perhaps we can buy some time for us to feel like everything is the way it used to be.

Gail is going to stop at the Cancer Center at lunch time on her way to a meeting downtown and will sit with him for a few minutes while Mom and Cathy get a bite to eat. This is going to be such a long, exhausting day for them. Dad, while hooked up, will be in a hospital bed and can nap if he feels like it. Mom and Cathy will be wandering and sitting in hospital chairs. I hope they don't have too many calls or visitors this evening. They were quite busy yesterday. People mean well but they just don't understand how difficult it is for Dad to pretend he is better than he actually is. He summons strength from somewhere and becomes a completely different person for the duration of their stay. I've seen it myself and commented to Dad that I hadn't realized just how tremendous a performance he was capable of giving. He said you can't let people see how you really feel when they take the time out of their day to visit. Once they leave he is absolutely drained.

I will call Gail this evening to hear how things went the rest of the afternoon.

I found Brandon in tears behind a tree last night when I went to say good night. He was sobbing uncontrollably and didn't want to tell me what it was all about nor did he want to be comforted by me. I'm certain he is feeling the stress and sadness I am feeling. He sees me crying from time to time. He feels things so deeply and hides it so the world doesn't know. Eventually, he made some feeble excuse about the source of his tears but I'm certain it is, in part at least, due to Dad's health and Brandon really doesn't know what is happening since they haven't seen Grandpa since early June and he still looked like Grandpa when we were there. I think we need to take the boys down this visit. I called to book Casper into the kennel for the weekend of August 20 and also asked about next week. She is available to keep him next week but is currently booked for the weekend. I don't know what we can do. Dad certainly can't have a dog in the house now that he is taking chemotherapy and we can't take him to Cathy's because of their dog. Patty is away that weekend or I'd ask her to keep him. I'm just stuck. I don't know what else to do.

Greg is terribly quiet and thoughtful. He asks everyday if I'd heard from Grandpa and Grandma. When I'm at Sharbot Lake and he is left at home the first thing he wants to know when I call home is about Grandpa. He wants to see what is going on but he is also afraid of what he will find out.

Last night I didn't have an appetite even though Ron made his famous spaghetti with meat sauce. I just picked at my plate. It tasted good but I just wasn't hungry. Ron took Casper for a walk while I cleaned up after dinner. I don't feel very social any more. Tonight I am going to suggest we visit Mike and Tracy as well as Cara over at the family cottage. Both she and Mel will be there this evening. I'm just afraid I'll break down into tears. I did that with Steve yesterday when he popped into visit me at the office. He told me I have the support of the entire Arnold family and I was to lean on them whenever I needed to. I try not to break down in front of people because that is hard on everyone and I don't want to put people in such an awkward position, especially when some people really don't know what to say to begin with. I have to try and summon some of the strength Dad is using when he has visitors.

## Thursday, July 28, 2005

***Mom*** and Dad called me last night. What an unexpected surprise. Mom sounded tired but in good spirits. She didn't know if I knew they had started Dad on his chemotherapy treatments. When I told her I had been in touch with Cathy and Gail a good part of the day she seemed surprised at first then realized she shouldn't have been. We beat the jungle drums often and loud!

After speaking to her for a few minutes Mom put Dad on the phone. He sounded much better than I had expected. He said, aside from feeling quite tired as he didn't sleep much the night before, he felt pretty good. Gail had brought him some chicken noodle soup in a thermos when she stopped by to sit with him at lunch time. He said he didn't think he wanted the soup but he did start to eat it and it tasted good to him so he finished the soup. In fact, the steroids must be working because he ate everything they had packed in the snack box; crackers, grapes, puddings, etc. Mom said Dad was into the cupboards when they got home and ate a good supper when it was ready. The nurse told him he may be "wired" for the evening because he had a lot of drugs in his system. Dad said he didn't think he was feeling "wired" but he's been feeling so poorly for so long that maybe "wired" feels the energetic way he used to feel. Dad didn't talk long but he told me a little bit about what they had done and when he started to feel tired he turned the phone backover to Mom. I told her they should try for an early night and turn on the answering machine. She thought that sounded like a good idea.

I called Gail just after nine o'clock last night as per our arrangement. She said the physical difference between how Dad was when he walked into the Cancer Center and how he was when he walked out made even his doctor stop and tell him how much better he looked. He had been hydrated for two hours which may have had a lot to do with how he looked and felt. The nurse told him most patients come back to their second treatment saying how well they have felt.

Gail also explained they planned to do six cycles of chemotherapy over the next three months with the hopes the tumors will shrink and any other cancer cells in his body are killed before they have time to do any damage. They will do radiation eventually but they want to keep that for future attacks.

He didn't hesitate when the doctor asked if he was prepared to begin his chemotherapy yesterday. "Yes!" he said, "Let's get started!"

I haven't heard how he is feeling this morning. Cathy usually drops in around 10am and stays until noon. She said she'd let Gail know how she found things and Gail can e-mail me. Yes, we communicate quite well! He can have soup for lunch and I'll know what kind it was ten minutes after he's eaten!

Gail is planning to go to Mom and Dad's Friday night to give Cathy a break. Mom and Dad don't require babysitting but it is nice to give Mom someone to visit with and Dad the support. Truthfully, it is for our benefit as well. Cathy, Gail and I all want to be with them as much as we can and since one keeps the others informed of how things are we're comfortable with taking turns. Bradley is turning sweet sixteen on Friday and is planning a party at the old farm house they recently purchased. Cathy and Steve both want to be around so they can control things a little. Gail thought if she went out Cathy wouldn't feel like she is torn between the two places and afraid she might miss a call from Mom. I think it is a great plan.

Ron and I are planning to go to Sharbot Lake next week for a couple of days and help Cathy and Steve do some of the work which needs to be done at the farm. There are beaver dams which need to be pulled-out to avoid pastures and roads from being flooded. The hedge needs to be trimmed and a few other chores are planned for when the extra manpower is there. We'll do what we can and Gail and Rob will help on the weekend. I'm not sure how long we will be able to stay. If we plan to be there through the week then Casper can go to the kennel. If we plan to stay past Friday then the kids can't come because the kennel is full and there isn't anyone who will be able to look after Casper.

## Tuesday, August 9, 2005

*I* didn't end up going to Sharbot Lake after all. I've had a very bad cold and because Dad has started chemotherapy his immune system is comprised and we must be careful not to knowingly bring germs into his environment. Ron, however, was feeling fine and he went to Sharbot Lake on Thursday and stayed at Cathy and Steve's.

Ron had a really good time with everyone and they got a lot of things accomplished at the farm. He and Steve went to the farm on Friday morning to begin trimming the cedar hedge. Cathy, Dad and Mom came up later and brought lunch with them. They had a few beer and some laughs. Dad ate a good lunch and then had a short nap. He didn't do any of the work but he did supervise the workers. Dad always says, "It's a poor job that can't afford one supervisor!"

Dad drove home and then he and Mom went out to Cathy's for a BBQ. I spoke to Ron just as Dad was about to have a piece of blueberry pie! In our family that's huge!! When Dad was growing up in the depression years he had to pick the tiny blueberries and then sell then for ten-cents a basket. The picking was hard work and since they were plentiful his mother would use them anyway she could in her cooking. As a result, Dad convinced himself he didn't like blueberries and during my entire lifetime I don't think I ever saw him eat any. So Ron really did witness something pretty special in our family's history!

On Saturday morning Ron, Steve and Cathy returned to the farm to pull out another beaver dam before Ron left for South River. In the same way I wish I was closer to help Mom, Dad and Cathy, Ron wishes he was closer to help Mom, Dad and Steve with whatever needs to be attended to. Ron arrived at our cottage around 5pm. I was eager to hear everything about Dad and Ron's time with my family. Ron told me Dad still looked frail but his voice sounded strong and his appetite is increasing everyday.

On Saturday evening Dad went with Steve to the farm and walked into where the beaver dams had been pulled apart. The hike through the bush would have been long for Dad but he obviously felt like going. So, we are all feeling much better about his progress so soon after he has begun his chemotherapy. He has had two treatments and will have this Wednesday off and begin the cycle again next week. His routine will be a long chemotherapy treatment followed, the next week, by a short treatment and then a rest week. This three week grouping makes one cycle.

ABC news anchor Peter Jennings died on Sunday night four months after announcing that he had lung disease. This news shook both Gail and I and, although I haven't spoken to Cathy, I'm sure she has heard the news and it affected her, too. His diagnosis came just three weeks ahead of Dad's. Today, on the news, it was announced that Dana Reeves, widow of Christopher Reeves, has also been diagnosed as having lung cancer. She is forty-seven years-old with a young son. I feel so sad for that little boy.

Gail and I were speaking last night and we have noticed subtle ways Dad is trying to prepare us for the inevitable separation. Their answering machine at home has always had Dad's voice on the machine telling the caller that, "Ethel and I can't come to the phone right now …" There is a new message, for no apparent reason, and it is Mom's voice that gives the message. He is beginning to make small changes, and I know him so well, all of these changes are well thought out. In the future, after he is gone, he doesn't want us to make a call and hear his voice even though, personally, I think I will cherish the sound of his voice for the rest of my life. He has also started to communicate less frequently via e-mail. Since he went on-line February 14, 2001 we have corresponded almost daily. Now, suddenly, even when he is starting to feel more energetic and have more interest in things he is sending only infrequent, brief e-mails.

During my conversation with Gail I made some reference to Dad's cancer being slow growing and hoping he has two to three good quality years. There was silence before Gail said that she didn't want to upset me but she felt a year was probably more realistic. In my heart this is something I've known but I try to fool myself into believing we won't have to deal with Dad's passing for some time yet. I still have waves of emotion washing over me but I'm moving more towards acceptance. Although, even when Dad actually passes, I feel certain it will still be a shock. I don't know how I'm ever going to get through the next few years. It just doesn't seem "do-able" to me.

Dad has two appointments today in Kingston. One is just to close the file with Dr Reid (the surgeon who talked him into the surgery) and the other is with Dr Kerr who is his eye specialist. Since Dad came home from the hospital he has had several broken blood vessels in his right eye. Dr Bell told him it could be cancer related or it could be from the retching or coughing or Cathy thinks it could be from dehydration when he first came home from the hospital. I suppose it could be anything and before Dr Bell treats it he wants the specialist to look at it which is, I think, a good plan. His appointment with Kerr was supposed to be at 2pm and it is now 2:50pm so I'm hoping to hear the outcome from Gail before I go home this afternoon or by phone tonight. She said she'd let me know one way or the other.

Our days seem to revolve around Dad's appointments and how he is feeling/eating/sleeping. I know we said at the onset that we would try to keep life as normal as possible for as long as possible, but I'm finding it hard to remember what was "normal". Everyone's voice seems to be a bit strained, our focus is on Dad's cancer, and we're all so sentimental and emotional in a reserved way. Words to songs I've heard a million times before will move me to tears and I've become terribly anxious. We seem to be more aware of news items pertaining to lung cancer. We've stopped making plans for the future. I can't remember when I last said, "Next week I'm going to …" Every happy situation is bitter sweet and there is a slight feeling of guilt that we are enjoying ourselves when Dad's health is so fragile. I don't think Dad's lung cancer is ever out of my mind. I haven't had the heart to entertain out at the cottage as we had planned to do. I just can't make any plans and summer is quickly disappearing.

I wrote to my uncle in Houston and tried to send a positive message to convey our family's unity and devotion and our strength. I told him Dad and Mom's spirits are good and when our family gets together we have a surprisingly good time with lots of laughter and trips down memory lane which is the way we've always handled family situations. Nobody is exempt from the unity of our circle and that gives us the strength which *is* our family.

Support has been forthcoming from some unexpected sources and these gestures, regardless how small, have the ability to lighten my day. We cling to every kindness, every gesture of comfort and will always remember it.

## Wednesday, August 10, 2005

*Dad's* eye doctor has never seen anything like the growth on his eye and feels it may be a secondary tumor. His wife is an ophthalmologist and she doesn't know what it is either so they have referred him to a specialist in this area. If it is a secondary tumor both doctors said these were rare. I'm not sure what to make of this. Shouldn't the chemotherapy be reducing this tumor? Wouldn't it have shown up during one of Dad's scans? If secondary tumors are starting to sprout does this mean we are further along in the process then we had expected?

Gail and I spoke for quite a while last night. Both of us felt deflated and numb. She had spoken to both Mom and Dad and after briefly mentioning the doctors' thoughts they both discussed other, upbeat family news. Bradley wrote his driver's test and passed so he will soon be sitting behind the wheel! They both didn't seem to want to talk about what this newest development might mean and Gail took her cue from them.

We spoke about how we are living day to day; hardly daring to breathe when things are going well because we have seen how quickly things can change. I was looking at my 2004 journal and saw I bought my first Christmas present a year ago next week. I can't even begin to think about Christmas. We just seem to be losing ground everyday. I just want to gather him into my arms and keep him safe just like he has always done for me. But, I can't do that this time. Everything is not OK and Dad already knows the depth of my emotions. He told me once that he and Mom know each of us as well as we know ourselves and I truly believe him. Over the years they have proved it over and over again. For me to totally break down with Dad would be his undoing and I won't be the one to add more pain to an already painful situation. I just keep thinking how Dad has been there for all the big and little events which make up a life; my life. I was his first-born. The child which made him a father but he loved Cathy and Gail no less because they arrived after me. We've always held our own special places in his heart. He was with me when I took my first steps. Mom and I met Dad at the kitchen door every evening when he returned from work. I would take his hand and toddle across the kitchen floor with my Dad. On this eventful, winter evening I took Dad's gloved hand and without my realizing he slipped his hand out of the glove and I continued across the kitchen stepping out on my own for the first time but carrying my Dad's faith in my abilities as I stepped proudly across the floor. His faith in me has continued to allow me to step out into the world and rise to new challenges.

I just received an e-mail from Dad and Mom. If anyone else read the e-mail they would never imagine, for even a minute, the situation we are dealing with. His letter was lengthy and chatty; just the way it always used to be. The letter seemed so "normal".

---

**Subject: Good morning!**
**Date:    2005 August 10—10:59**

From:   Harold Clark
To:     Susan Arnold

Hi, Susan

I thought we would beat you to the computer this morning. Very nice day here; bright sunshine and warm, too. We had not too bad of a day yesterday. We saw Dr. Reid, the surgeon, who was satisfied with his end of things. Then, on to Dr. Kerr who examined my eye. He thinks it is related to my problem, however, he said it was beyond his expertise and is forwarding me to his specialist just in case. He gave me some drops to help in the meantime.

Bradley got his drivers test so he is happy; now we'll all have to stay off the road!! Everything else is fine here. Mom keeps me well fed and watered so there is nothing that can be complained about.

How is your cold coming along? Are you taking care of it or just letting it go (shame on you). How are Ron and the boys?

Nothing else here so I'll sign off and get to work. Have a good day. Say Hi to all and we'll be in touch.

Love Mom and Dad

We had a bad wind and rain storm last night which knocked-out the hydro in the village and at the lake, as well as knocking the water treatment plant offline. As a result we had to go to a Water Advisory and then to a Boil Water Advisory as a precautionary measure as mandated by provincial regulations.

I'm heading to North Bay after work this evening. Sometimes the only thing which will help me feel better is to spend money! I don't know what I'm going to shop for but I'm not leaving there until I've pulled out my American Express card! Maybe I'll find the perfect dress to wear to Andrea's wedding and for many other events later. I'd like something classic and a bit unusual.

## Thursday, August 11, 2005

*Well*, my shopping trip seems to have been a success. I found some black chiffon panel pants and a dusty rose and black crepe top which I can wear with gold jewellery and a string of pink pearls and I'll carry my black evening bag. I think it will look very stylish. I'm not looking forward to this wedding as much as I was a year ago when Andrea told us they were engaged. I guess everything is relative and Dad's health just effects how I view everything.

I had a really good sleep last night; the first in weeks. I don't remember Ron leaving for the store this morning at his usual 4:30am. Normally, I would be aware of his moving around the cottage and hear the door close but I heard nothing this morning. My arthritis seems to be flaring up a bit. Last night both my wrists and hands began to swell and become sore. Pushing open a door or driving the car was painful. They are somewhat better today but I think it is the stress which is bringing on this flare up. I'll just rest them and take some anti-inflammatory tablets.

The sun is out today and things seem to be quiet around the village which is nice after yesterday's water troubles and the storm's aftermath. I think last night was good for me to get out alone and look at all the new fall fashions and accessories. I've always had an interest in fashion and like to see what's "in" for the next season.

When I reread entries in this journal it sometimes looks as though I'm always on the verge of tears. In actual fact, there are twenty-four hours in each day and to most of the world I look like I'm coping pretty well. These entries are how I'm feeling on the inside.

I sigh a lot, lately.

I e-mailed both Gail and Dad this morning but, as yet, I've heard nothing back from either of them. Things seem so strange. I go to work, throw laundry into the machine, talk to people about the Village's budget and try to continue on but I feel like I'm looking through very dark glasses. It's like the sun has been erased. Mom mentioned "the hole in our hearts" the end of May and I guess that is an appropriate description. Things which used to have meaning don't have any meaning now. I would like to think I will handle all of this with a dignity and a composure which will make Dad proud of me. Even now, at the age of forty-six, I still have the desire to make Dad and Mom proud in some form or another. Truthfully, I know, without a doubt, they are proud of me and the life I have built with Ron. They believe in all of us and they truly enjoy spending time together with my sisters and I and our families. We like each other and have common interests. When I look ahead into the future I guess I'll miss Dad's friendship, his sense of humor and his wisdom the most. I don't need a father to tuck me into bed at nights or discipline me or tell me what I need to do but I do need my friend to laugh with, to travel with, to gossip with and to enjoy life with. I need my friend to confide in, to lean upon, to run ideas past and to connect with my heritage. I don't think there is a day in his life when he doesn't learn something. He follows local, national and international news and is very aware of economic, environmental and political events and how they effect our family. His interest in life and his passion for living life is one of the qualities I've admired for longer than I can remember and spending any amount of time with him makes everyone feel that excitement and interest in life.

He taught me to collect experiences and memories. He's someone who appreciates a picnic along the road as well as a meal at a five star restaurant. He's stayed in a tent and stayed in top notch resorts. He's been a member of the head table and then came home, changed into his brown overalls and went out to rake the leaves in the back yard. He's a man who has remained curious. Even now, he asks questions about the medical equipment the doctors use to track his illness. Some people stop learning when they leave school. Dad has never stopped learning. He is a very intelligent, educated man who can ask questions which can, and have, stumped people with impressive educational degrees. God certainly blessed Dad from the day of his birth, with talents he has used to create a life full of love, interest and colour.

## Friday, August 12, 2005

*Gail* and I had another lengthy discussion last night via the phone. The Bell Canada Phone Company is certainly happy we are their customers! She has been experiencing a similar week to mine. She has been very fragile and struggles everyday to maintain some composure so her colleagues don't catch her in tears. She hasn't any patience and everyone seems to be on her last nerve. I know those feelings so well and I believe it helps both of us to vent and wallow and keep the lines of communication open. We are both aware of what the other is going through. I cherish our ability to share so much with each other. We've always been able to talk about our joys, triumphs, disappointments and now, our sorrow. We always seem to be "in tune" with one another.

I just called Mom and Dad's and Dad answered the phone. He sounded good and was busy visiting with Cathy and Steve. He asked about the store, about Ron and the boys and about the remnants my cold before passing the phone over to Mom. Mom sounded tired. Even now that Dad sleeps during the night I don't think Mom sleeps well. I think, in the dark, Mom looks into the future and sheds her tears when there isn't anyone else around. Unlike the rest of us, Mom can't really express the depth of her sadness without making it harder on Dad who really only gets upset when one of us cries or gets choked up. The rest of us can cry and be comforted by our spouses but Mom really can't do that until Dad is sleeping. She must feel very lonely at times.

Rob had made me a disc of digital pictures from Panama, the farm and Gail's graduation. I couldn't bring myself to look at them until today. We had such a great time in Panama! Seeing the pictures brought back so many memories and none of them made me cry. We looked happy and relaxed and Rob also took pictures of many aspects of Panama life which is also nice to have. As I viewed the pictures I wrote down the ones I'd like to have enlarged or printed off to put into our scrapbook. The ones of our family of four turned out really well. The two pictures of the "original five" and the entire family are good, too, so I see several framing opportunities. There is also a picture of Cathy, Gail and I that I'd like to have framed. Until now, my office has only had pictures of Ron and the boys. I think I'll add a few extras. I also want several of the Panama pictures to frame and put at the cottage. Rob did a great job.

Gail and I talked last night about getting something extra special for Cathy and Steve to commemorate their twentieth wedding anniversary. We feel they have shouldered extra responsibilities since Dad's illness and they deserve to be fussed over. We want to help in any way we can but logic says it is easier for Cathy to drive them to an appointment then for Ron and I to come to drive them. Cathy doesn't mind but it is still tiring for her. She never complains and I've told her to call and Ron or I or both of us will be there. Ron went down last week to help and they plan to do a few other things when we return on August 19. Cathy and I have talked so many times on the phone since Dad's diagnosis. She appears strong and courageous to the world but I worry about her, too, because she's so close in proximity to Mom and Dad and it will be very hard for her as Dad's cancer progresses. She can't escape reality the way Gail or I can. I hope she talks to Steve to get a lot of her feelings out into the open. It just isn't good for her health to hold all these conflicting emotions inside. I respect her right to privacy and won't press her. When she's ready to talk, and if she wants me, I'll be there to listen. She is so strong, yet when I look at her I can still see my little sister whose heart would break when she saw a stray kitten or a robin with a broken wing. Cathy was given to me as a birthday present when she was born four days before my birthday and came home from the hospital on the day I turned two years-old. How many little girls get a real, live baby for a birthday gift? To me, the confident, independent, capable woman who takes care of everyone around her will remain my special birthday present, my eager playmate and my willing partner-in-crime! And, like all special gifts I want to take very good care of her.

I have been reading a book about Jackie Onassis and how she handled herself when John Kennedy died, when her half-sister died of lung cancer and then the months and days leading to her own death. Much of what has been written shows enormous dignity and strength and an acceptance of God's Will. She looked at life in much the same way Dad looks at life regarding what is important. They both placed a tremendous value on family and living life to its fullest. I hope someone will be able to say the same about me when I pass from this world.

Cara, our niece, and her friends are arriving at the Arnold family cottage tonight. I look forward to seeing her and perhaps discussing our hot air balloon adventure. I know it sounds silly but it is definitely something I want to do and I can't for the life of me explain why! I'm afraid of heights! I would love to share the experience with Dad and Mom byway of pictures and tales from above the earth. Dad's illness has really impressed upon me the need to never put something off which is important to us. I've tried to live that way. I've always said I'll be dead a lot longer than I'll be alive. I've tried to teach the boys to collect memories and experiences from a very early age. We've done some amazing things. The one thing which seems to stand out in their memories is the day I woke them up and suggested we play "hooky". The boys neither knew what hooky was nor believed me when I told them we weren't going to go to school or work and, instead, we were going on a picnic. They still talk about that day!

Tracy and Mike and their children, Derek and Lauren, arrived at their cottage yesterday afternoon. Mike is Ron's first cousin and they own a cottage near ours. Ron was into my office an hour ago and wondered about inviting them over for pizza and beer. I said that would be great especially since today is cold (seventeen degrees) and rainy so they may want to get out of the cottage and come for a visit. We enjoy spending time with them. Our kids have become very close but then, they've spent a good part of every summer together at the family cottage since they were small babies.

So, for the moment, our emotional storms seem to have passed and we are preparing for a normal weekend at the cottage. Things could change by tomorrow but for now, things are pretty good and we have to find blessings where we can.

## Monday, August 15, 2005

*We* did have a good weekend. Tracy and Mike and the kids did come over on Friday. They were at the cottage when I got home after work. We had a nice visit. Next morning, Ron made my coffee and we sat outside enjoying the morning. We rounded up all the garbage and he made a trip into town, stopping at the landfill site on his way. I did several loads of laundry and then, after lunch, Ron and Greg headed to Bracebridge, Ontario, a resort town to the south of South River. The Triple 'A' hockey try-outs for the Orillia Minor Midgets were this weekend. They also went down on Sunday but, in the end, both he and his friend, Brody, were selected as APs (alternate players). They were very disappointed and I feel badly for Greg. He tried to make himself believe he wouldn't be chosen but deep down it meant a lot to him to be selected. Ron said he'd call North Bay and see if they've picked their Triple 'A' team.

Our Sunday morning was interrupted early when a friend of Ron's called at 8am to ask Ron if he'd play in a ball tournament at 9:30am. The team had two injuries on Saturday and needed another player. Ron really didn't want to go but he agreed and was home again around noon. Brandon stayed at his friend's, D J Wainman, on Saturday night. I miss him so much when he is away. He has such sparkle and makes every day so exciting. Sometimes this very trait is enough to try my patience but when I really think about it, this is what makes Brandon so special. He has a taste for life and needs to be doing things constantly. He has often reminded me of Dad.

I went over to the family cottage for a short visit with Cara on Sunday morning. She isn't sure when she'll be back to South River. She's going to look into hot air ballooning for us.

Mom and Dad called just after Ron arrived back from playing ball and we had a nice chat. Dad sounds so strong and, for the first time since the end of April, we didn't talk about his illness or Doctor's appointments or even how he was feeling. He told us about going to Perth, about being at Bradley's ball tournament and about going to the church bake sale. He asked questions about the boys and how we were feeling and what we were doing. It was a very normal conversation that, somehow, now seems abnormal. After hanging up I felt sad. Yes, Dad is feeling well and he has resumed many of his normal activities but the summer is winding down and they haven't been here to visit the cottage and I feel his absence keenly. I can't wait until Thursday to see everyone. I have a hair appointment tonight so I'll look my best.

I heard from Dad and Mom via e-mail this afternoon. They sound busy and happy and that makes me pleased. I haven't heard anything from Gail but Cathy sent a little "funny" to give us our morning chuckle!

I think, sometime in September, I'm going to make an appointment with my doctor. I force myself to do things on a daily basis. I'd rather just fold my hands in my lap and stare at the lake. I don't look into the future and don't make any plans beyond today. I used to be full of plans. When I smile I feel like it is only my mouth. The smile doesn't go anywhere near my eyes or my heart. I find myself withdrawing into myself and seeking quiet solitude to remember, to think and to relive memories. Well meaning people ask me several times every day how Dad is and each time I say, "He's coming along" but I really want to scream and tell them, "there is no cure for lung cancer! My father is dying!" I want to rip the cigarette or pipe out of every person I see on the street! "What are you doing?" I'd like to yell at them. "Do you want your children to watch you die?" There is an anger held deep within me. If I'm not feeling better by the end of September I'll make my appointment and hope my doctor will give me a magical little pill to take away this sadness or numb the pain or just make the world make sense again.

## Tuesday, August 16, 2005

---

Subject: Re: Good Morning
Date:    2005 August 16—13:08
From:  Harold Clark
To:      Susan Arnold

Hi, Susan;

It is another nice day and the forecast calls for more this week; we'll take all we can get!!

Yes, Gail is coming out tonight and is going to keep me honest while I get my "fix" tomorrow. She wants to give Cathy a break so they can celebrate their anniversary. It sure doesn't seem like twenty years but it definitely is, like the old saying, "Time sure flies".

Mom has been doing her usual inside and I have finished the wheelbarrow project and I'm working on servicing the lawn tractor in the garage.

I suppose the boys are starting to get anxious about hockey camp and school and all the things they will be starting before long.

Nothing else here to talk about so I'll get back at it. Say Hi to all and we will be talking to you later.

Love Mom and Dad

Patty told me my hair looks really good but I can't say I'm really happy with it. The colour, in my opinion, is too dark for this time of year but I guess it is better than the grey roots which were showing. I feel bloated today, too As much as I enjoy the cottage I wonder if maybe we shouldn't stay at the house through the week and just go to the cottage on the weekends. My whole perspective seems so negative. I know a big part of how I'm feeling is because of Dad's health. The other part is my annual autumn doldrums. I can't make plans and winter, with its hockey schedules and its cold weather and Dad's cancer, seems to be crushing me from all sides. I realize I should be happy for the things I have. I keep telling myself to look for blessings where I can find them but the end of summer has always been a melancholy time for me.

### Wednesday, August 17, 2005

Today is Cathy and Steve's 20th wedding anniversary. Where has the time gone? Gail, Mom and Dad went out to visit them last night and to take them their gifts. We (Gail and my family) gave them a gift certificate to Minos, a Greek restaurant, which is in two locations in Kingston, and both Cathy and Steve enjoy the food that is served. They can either go alone or take the kids.

I called Ron to see if we should book an extra night at the hotel in Ottawa. He said he'd be OK with whatever I decide. Staying in Ottawa, shopping there and then heading home to South River would be easier. I don't remember much about the Bayshore Shopping Centre or the stores in it but I'm sure we'll find school shopping fun when we're shopping someplace different. Dad has chemotherapy today and we'll see how he is on the weekend. If he's doing well we may just stay in Ottawa leave for South River from there. If he's not feeling great we may come back to Sharbot Lake on Sunday to see him. I'm getting better at not making plans.

The boys have stayed in Ottawa several times. Twice as a family … this being the third time … and Brandon was there once with Ron on a school trip.

I was just speaking to Cathy at length. I called to wish her a Happy Anniversary. Steve won't be home until 6pm so they thought they'd just go to the restaurant at the Sharbot Lake Hotel and have dinner tonight and save their certificate for another time.

Gail has taken Dad and Mom to Dad's chemotherapy today. This is the first one of his second cycle so it is expected to be five to six hours just to let the drugs drip through his system. That's not counting the time for blood work and making up the drug cocktail. So, it is always a long day. Cathy wondered if I might take a turn since they'd been told the doctor expected Dad to have four to six cycles. I'm so pleased she asked if I would. I keep telling them we are available to help but Cathy keeps saying it is too far for us to drive for only one day. I don't mind. The week we have decided on is the 7th of September. I can leave after work on the Tuesday and be there in the early evening.

I told Cathy that as much as I love Mom and Dad I find visiting them very difficult. I told her I find it hard to go there and stay upbeat. It takes so much out of me. She can pop into their place, put on a good face and pop out again. When I'm there it is a constant act for at least two nights and I'm emotionally drained when I leave. Cathy says that Dad feeds off the upbeat, positive vibrations he gets from all of us, so if I can keep it up then so much the better but she understands how it must be. I'll do anything if it helps Dad and Mom.

I've tried screaming and punching a pillow but nothing really helps get this anger out of my system. It is the anger and the helplessness of the whole situation which keeps eating away at me. I have certainly gained a new appreciation for people who are losing relatives in a long battle with a disease. Knowing how much I care for my family I always thought the worst would be after their passing. I never dreamed a person is so affected by a disease in so many aspects of life. I think this journal has allowed me to express emotions and feelings I might not have been able to get any sort of a handle on without writing it down. I suppose it could be said that I'm obsessed with Dad's illness. I'm letting the cancer spread through me by allowing it to drain away my will to live life to its fullest. I'm allowing it to blacken the days, weeks and months I have with Dad. It's easy to say, but, oh, so hard to deal with in reality. I know pretending is stressful and exhausting. I wonder if maybe I shouldn't make plans for the future and give myself permission to look ahead. Dad has always lived his life by planning but also by letting the spirit move him. I know there were times when Mom and Dad would wake up on a cold winter's morning and decide to book a trip somewhere warm. They planned so they had the ability to travel at a moment's notice. Maybe I really should start remembering everything my parents taught me. This is life. The part of life which sucks but everyone has to go through it at some point or another. Our boys will have to bury us someday and life will continue. The sun will still rise and school will still be in session and someone's day will still have a couple of bumps in it and the traffic on Toronto's streets will still be backed-up at rush hour. Hard to imagine but how many funerals have we attended and then, after drying our tears, returned to the rituals of daily life? If we've been born into this world then we'll have to die to leave it and in between we will live. Those are the facts and it is what we choose to do with our life that counts.

# Thursday, August 18, 2005

***Ron*** and I took the boys to see the movie "The Dukes of Hazzard" and we enjoyed it more than I thought we would. I knew the boys would like it. Who wouldn't like fast cars and skimpy-dressed girls? The movie had a storyline that I was surprised to find we could follow. Everyone was in a good mood. We stopped at the mall and bought Brandon's dress pants and a few other things we needed and were back in the car twenty five minutes after leaving it. Good job! We went to the movie theater and discovered the movie started at 7:20 and not at 7pm so we had a few minutes breathing room. Ron bought our tickets and then ordered a pizza while the boys played in the arcade. I took a walk through the mall. We had fun and were home by 10pm. Ron and the boys gave Casper a bath while I sorted out what we needed to pack. It felt good to laugh and enjoy myself. I actually didn't consciously think about Dad for the first time in a long time.

This morning didn't get off to a great start. The boys were tired and it is their day to work at our store so I had to wait for them and was almost late getting to work myself. Brandon doesn't like what he's wearing to the wedding. He says he looks like a little kid. I think he looks handsome. He has his new black dress pants, shiny dress shoes, black belt, grey dress shirt, a wine colored tie and a black vest. He thinks the vest makes him look like a little kid. So, Ron is going to look for a men's small sports jacket today when he takes Casper to the kennel at North Bay. I look around and see what I need to do at lunchtime and the pressure starts to takeover. I really hate mornings like this.

I called Sharbot Lake this morning. I was afraid to pickup the phone in case Dad wasn't responding well to yesterday's treatment although, if he wasn't, it would be the first time. Mom answered and she said the day had gone well even though it had been a very long day. She said Dad got up this morning and ate a good breakfast and was just having a coffee and a granola bar when I called. The doctor said Dad had gained another pound which is good news. Dad said he is only three pounds lighter then he was when he stopped smoking five years ago.

I'm looking forward to a good weekend. We're all planning to go to the farm on Friday to get some work done for Dad. Ron and Steve plan to fix some fence posts and do some trimming. They'll likely want to check the beaver dams and make sure they haven't been rebuilt. Dad mentioned loading some wood onto a trailer and bringing it to Sharbot Lake for this winter. That's something the boys and I can work at. We're supposed to have a picnic lunch and I must remember to bring down the things I said I would. Cathy and Mom are taking care of the meat and buns. I'll bring cheese, carrots, dip, broccoli and cauliflower (good cancer-fighting vegetables) grapes, watermelon and perhaps a pineapple. That should fill the gap after working for the morning. Cathy said we'd BBQ something at their place for dinner on Friday night. Hopefully Gail and Rob will be able to join us.

Greg just called, bless his heart, he tries so hard to help me and I don't always appreciate what he does. He doesn't make his bed or pick up after himself without being told but he does help when he knows I'm counting on him. He is also very good at sitting quietly beside me and keeping me company. He and Brandon are going to pickup their things from the livingroom and pack their suitcases with clothes they need for the farm and what they want to wear while we are in Ottawa shopping for school supplies. I told him I'd take care of the wedding clothes. They are also going to put the dishes into the dishwasher. Then Greg plans to go to the gym to workout before we go away. When I get home at lunchtime I'll pack my things and iron their shirts. That shouldn't take my whole lunch-hour. Everything I need to pack is pretty much sitting where I can see it. Ron is taking Casper to North Bay. Hopefully we'll be on the road by 5:00pm. Maybe we can pack a few things to snack on so we don't have to stop on the way. Everyone goes to bed so early at both Mom and Dad's and at Cathy's. I'd hate to get in really late and disrupt everyone's schedule. Anyway, things seem to be getting done.

## Wednesday, August 24, 2005

***Dad*** had been quite well on Thursday when we arrived at Sharbot Lake. In fact, he was like a different man who came out to the kitchen to greet us. He had put on some weight and had colour in his skin. His voice was strong and he seemed to have energy even though it was the day after his heavy dose of chemo. They were tired from their previous day at the hospital. Dad, because of stimulates in the chemotherapy, doesn't sleep much the night following his treatment so he was ready for bed about 9:30. We all were.

Friday morning we were up bright and early and, when Cathy and Steve arrived at 8:30am, we were ready to head to the farm, at Arden. There were a lot of projects which needed to be done and Dad would be very happy with whatever we accomplished. As soon as we arrived, shortly after 9:00am, and unloaded the food hampers, coolers and implements we needed to do our assorted jobs we got started. Ron and Steve had to replace five fence posts with cedar posts which had been cut previously. There was wood to load into the back of Steve's truck and the attached trailer which Cathy, Mom, Greg and Brandon got busy with. Later, the boys took the four-wheeler and brought the fence posts to where Ron and Steve were working. I was on the lawn tractor cutting the grass. The yard is huge and took several hours. The boys took turns with the whip-per-snipper around the buildings. Mom and Cathy were busy in the kitchen keeping ahead of the hungry workers! Lunch was terrific! Lunch meat, buns, cheeses, fruit, vegetables, pickles; everything anyone could want. Back to work after lunch. The guys all went to check the beaver dams and ended up pulling two apart. Dad had a small lie down after lunch but I think he enjoyed getting out and about with everyone. Once everything was done we had some cold drinks before heading back to Sharbot Lake. Everyone pitched in and unloaded the cord of wood we had brought from the farm. With all hands on deck it took forty minutes to unload, carry down to the basement and stack the wood we had brought with us. Mom and Dad don't depend on wood to keep warm but they do enjoy a wood fire and Dad finds it a more warming heat so he has been put-ting wood in the stove more often the past couple of years. After the work was done it was party time! Unfortunately, by this time, Dad was suffering with an intense pain in his sternum which has become a frequent problem since his surgery. The doctors feel it is likely "mechanical". The pain is very intense and completely floors him. His colour becomes very pale and heat seems to help. Yet, when it is over, like a kidney or gall stone passing, the pain is gone and, aside from being tired, he is ready to eat his dinner. Fortunately, the pain left shortly before we began to BBQ around 7pm. Cathy and Mom really went all out once again, but that is what we grew up with … lots of food, well prepared and served with love and laughter. And Saturday's meal wasn't any different. Dad and I sat in the dining room and he ate a good meal and chatted about all sorts of things. To look at him I found it hard to believe he is so ill. The boys noticed Grandpa had lost some weight but they didn't see any other changes which I found comforting. Dad was so happy about all the tasks we had gotten done at the farm. He can't think of another thing which needs to be done to prepare it for winter aside from, perhaps, one more grass-cutting. Having someone else do the jobs that Dad would ordinarily do is very hard on him and he becomes quite humble, proud and grateful when we pull together and do the jobs for him.

The boys went to Cathy's for the night. They showered at her place in the morning to cut down on bathroom traffic getting ready for the wedding. I hated to leave; especially since Dad's chest pain had returned and he was stretched out on the couch waiting for the pain to subside. He was able to be in the kitchen as we headed out the door. We didn't make any promises about returning on Sunday but, given how he was feeling, Ron and I both felt we would be back.

The wedding was lovely. The boys took it all in but, in the end, decided they didn't want to attend the reception. They'd had enough "dress up" although they did look so tall and handsome. The next morning I was awake ahead of everyone else and went downstairs to the Tim Horton's Coffee Shop on the first floor of the hotel and bought an assortment of drinks and pastries for our breakfast. We called Dad and Mom and learned Dad was feeling much better. He'd had some rest Saturday afternoon and the pain had left and hadn't returned. Gail had given him an antacid. We're not sure if acid is the cause of the pain or if the attack had merely run its course. So, feeling as though things were good at Mom and Dad's we decided to stay in Ottawa and return to South River from there on Monday.

We had a great day! After getting ready we headed out to explore the Nation's Capital on foot. Brandon and Ron had been to Ottawa on a school trip in June last year but, usually, the boys have only visited Ottawa in the winter when everything is cold, snow covered and icy. The day was warm and sunny and perfect for exploring. We walked to the pedestrian street known as The Spark's Street Mall. This street is closed to vehicle traffic and has lots of outdoor cafes and bistros. We walked to the Rideau Center and shopped for a while before having our lunch there. Then we walked along the Rideau Canal with all the boats bobbing next to their moorings. We took several pictures of the boys and our family with the canal and the Ottawa landmarks in the background. We didn't arrive back to our room until after 5pm. We had a short nap and then Ron and Greg went for a swim in the hotel pool while Brandon and I watched some TV. When the guys came back we walked to a Mexican restaurant for our dinner. The food was good, the decor looked authentic and Greg decided to try deep fried ice cream for dessert. After walking back the boys went up to our room and Ron and I continued for a walk around a few more blocks. It had been a wonderful day. We watched a movie and then turned in for the night with a promise to get up at a reasonable hour to check out and head to the Bayshore Shopping Center to shop for school clothes.

Next day, without getting lost, we arrived at the mall around 10am and began to make our purchases. Around 2pm we headed for South River arriving there at 6pm. I felt like I'd been away for two weeks. The change of routine and scenery had done me a lot of good. I felt relaxed and really hadn't concentrated on Dad's health. The boys had been great. We enjoyed the time we had been together having fun and seeing things we don't see everyday. It was a mini-vacation that the whole family enjoyed. While we had shopped I found a London Fog all-weather coat and a sweater set and a few other little trinkets to brighten my fall wardrobe. I picked up a couple of books which were on sale and the boys were decked out top-to-toe with their new school clothes. They were very pleased with their purchases and thanked us many times. Before long we were back at the cottage and happy to be there.

I spoke to both Dad and Mom when we returned on Monday evening. They sounded very good and Dad hadn't experience any return of his chest pain. They'd had some company over the weekend but not enough to tire them out. He spent Monday in his workshop at the end of the garage servicing his weed-eater.

Yesterday was nice, a little chilly perhaps, but still very nice. After work the boys and I went out to the cottage and Ron stayed in town to play baseball. This was the second game out of a three game play-off. They have won both games. The final is on Thursday. I prepared the boys tacos and a salad for dinner while I enjoyed an omelet and salad. I went for a twenty minute walk and when I returned Greg asked me to go kayaking with him. The water was calm and the evening was perfect for drifting along. We talked a lot. Greg wanted to know about Grandma Arnold. He was only seven when she died and he seems to feel he is losing her in his memories. I told him stories about her and by the end of the paddle he knew she was still a very strong memory and that made him feel much better. We talked about grade ten and the courses he will be taking. We watched a loon who swam close to us and then, when it saw us, let out a war-hoop! It was a great evening. I like getting the boys by themselves for some time with me. After we returned he, Brandon and Casper disappeared into the bunkhouse to play one of their new video games and I cleaned up the kitchen before sitting down to read one of my new books. Ron got home around 10pm.

Today is Dad's moderate treatment. He said they hoped to have his blood work done by 9am and have his doctor's appointment at 10:30am so they could begin his treatment on schedule. I think he said the treatment was scheduled for 1pm. After they finish they are planning to go to Gail's and stay the night. He has an appointment with an eye specialist tomorrow to determine what this thing on his iris really is. The other doctor felt it may be cancer-related and even a secondary tumor. Perhaps the chemotherapy will have reduced the tumor, if in fact that is what it is, as I thought his eye looked quite a bit better when I saw him. Anyway, we are anxious to get the finally word on this latest development and what, if anything, can be done about it.

So, that is where we sit for today. Things are progressing nicely and, Dad's spirits seem to be staying up which is beneficial on its own. As difficult a time as I've had keeping my emotions in check I am still amazed at how matter-of-fact Dad has been through all of this. He definitely hasn't given-up. He keeps saying we'll beat this thing. I also believe, when Dad gets quiet and withdraws, he is recharging the energy he needs to fight the disease. He is carefully weighing everything he has been told to be sure he understands each step of the cancer-fighting process. If there is anything he can do to fight the cancer he will but he has also said he'll know when to let nature take its course. I had a small moment this morning for the first time in a couple of weeks but the moment passed and I'm fine.

## Thursday, August 25, 2005

*I* spoke to Gail last night. She seemed pleased with how Dad's appointment went yesterday. There was a different doctor filling-in for Dr Gregg, Dad's oncologist, but they liked her very much. She was bubbly yet professional. She was happy with how Dad was progressing with his treatments. She gave him a prescription for some pills to take in the morning which are more antacid then anti-nausea. The Dr. feels Dad's pain is definitely acid reflux or overactive acid which has been bothering him. It began after he was in the hospital and receiving quite a few different types of medications and the lining of his gastric system has likely been irritated before he began chemotherapy treatments and now the chemotherapy is effecting it. Dad mentioned that the antacid tablets seemed to help so the doctor is even more certain that acid is the cause. So, he'll give this a try. I hope this helps as the pain takes him completely off his feet and really wipes him out after the attack. Dad also lost about half a pound since last week but, as he says, because of the pain in his chest he really didn't feel much like eating so he felt it was reasonable to have dropped a bit of weight.

Mom and Dad were very pleased with how quickly things at the Cancer Clinic moved along yesterday. Dad was actually finished his treatment and leaving the hospital fifteen minutes before his chemotherapy appointment was scheduled to begin. So, Gail, Mom and Dad went back to her house, had a bite to eat and a little rest. Then they did some errands. Later, they lounged in chairs outside at Gail's. Everyone sounded to be in good spirits and I was happy to end the call on that note.

Dad and Mom drove themselves into Kingston yesterday morning so my coming down to "take" them to chemotherapy won't fly with Dad. I've already decided I'll just tell them I would like to go with them and see the process for myself. Everyone else has been there and I'd like to go, too. I think that will pacify both Dad and Mom.

Cathy is going to give me a call tonight to tell me how things go at Dad's appointment with the eye specialist this afternoon. Dad's health seems to be stable and we're adjusting very well. Cathy didn't go with Dad and Mom for his treatment this week because Gail is on vacation and she wanted to go with them. Dad doesn't have chemotherapy next week and the following Wednesday I will be there so Cathy will have a break for at least four weeks. She had been steady on the road for appointments and tests from the very beginning. I'm glad she will have time to do some of the other things Cathy likes to do. This morning she is making pickles and relish. Cathy is very domestic and likes to do this kind of thing but normally doesn't have the luxury of time as she is usually working. She is so relaxed and contented at present despite the turmoil we've been going through.

I've been busy at the office but I think I'm getting everything done which is a priority. The big thing is the tax bills which need to go into the mail next week. Once they are out then I can start on my list of "catch up work" so my desk stays current. I would like to have this desk in good shape in case I need to leave suddenly. In the same way, I'd like to have things kept up to-date at home just because Mom and Dad may need some help for the autumn cleanup and I'd like to be free to go if they call and not feel guilty that my own stuff is going behind. I may even need to stay later at work from time to time just to make sure my work gets completed. I don't want to take advantage of the Village's understanding and goodwill.

## August 29, 2005

*It's* been two years ago today since Ron and I bought our family cottage. It was a big investment but it has given us so much pleasure already. We said when we bought it that we wanted it to be a retreat for our family to spend time together and reconnect. It has been that and more. The cottage has been a place for family and friends and, this year, it has been a place to recharge and gain my balance in the face of many emotional storms due to Dad's illness. The cottage is a place where we can spend one-on-one time with the boys and let them see us as individuals as well as their parents and it is a place Ron and I can be a couple. We take pleasure in sharing a coffee/tea under the maple trees or a walk along Scarlett Road. We look forward to quiet kayak rides after dinner and going for swims. It has become a place where we can talk about anything and make plans for the day/week/month ahead. It has truly become "our place." The four of us have already accumulated many wonderful memories at our cottage.

Dad's eye appointment went well, all things considered. The doctor took a number of tests and an ultrasound of the small one-millimeter tumor. She feels it is a cancer tumor but wants all the relative data from these tests as well as the file from Dad's cancer doctor before making an absolute determination. I like that strategy. Too many times now the doctors blurt out the first thing they think regardless of what that does to the patient and the family. She also wants to confer with a colleague in Toronto as tumors on the iris are quite rare. She wants to see how deep it goes and what feeds it. Then they can determine how to treat it. They plan to see Dad in two weeks. That may just work well with my schedule to be with them.

I called Mom and Dad on Friday morning and they seemed to be doing fine. Cathy and Steve had arrived to visit and Cathy was organizing Dad's newest pills. There is quite an assortment on the kitchen counter. For a man who seldom took an aspirin he certainly has a number of pill bottles with his name on them.

When we spoke on Sunday they sounded rested and quite normal. In fact, they had been out to church in the morning which was the first time they'd been back since the Sunday before Dad's surgery in June. They found it difficult being the center of attention. Everyone was shaking Dad's hand and the ladies were kissing him. He said he felt like the most important man in Sharbot Lake! But then, we always knew that!! He and Steve are planning to go fishing in the late afternoon. Mom is going to go to Cathy's and they'll all have dinner together tonight. Sounds like a nice day planned.

Ron spoke to Steve and they made plans for Ron to go to Sharbot Lake on Wednesday after work to help Steve for a couple of days catch-up on bringing his winter wood in and any other little projects he needs to do before the cold weather arrives. We're trying to start some of our autumn chores in between trips to Sharbot Lake. Ron will return on Saturday. Dad and Mom seemed disappointed that we weren't coming with Ron although they always love seeing him, too. So, I told them I was coming down the following Tuesday to go into Kingston with them for Dad's chemotherapy. Dad said that wasn't necessary and I said it was. I told them I wanted to see what it was all about and I've already cleared my schedule. Mom said the day will be long but she'd be happy to have me there for company. Dad finally agreed and I think the matter is settled. They don't want to feel they are a burden and I said to Cathy there are things in life we *have* to do and things in life we *want* to do. Dad *has* to take chemotherapy treatments and I *want* to be there for him.

I was pleased yesterday when we spoke to Mom and Dad. They said they'd like to come to South River for a weekend before we close up the cottage to see all the painting we've done and have a visit. Even if we weren't staying at the cottage they'd still like to visit. Naturally, I'd be thrilled to get them here. Their absence from the cottage this summer has been a real bruise on my heart. Perhaps Cathy and Steve can bring Mom and Dad here and spend the weekend with us. I know Dad is quite capable of driving shorter distances but, our place is so far, and what if he has a wave of fatigue or that acid reflux? The drive would take too much out of them. I find it nerve wracking by times and I drive it often so I'm certain they'd find it even more so. I'd be so delighted to look out the window at the cottage and see Dad getting out of the car.

Dad just e-mailed me. He has been in his workshop servicing the outboard motor most of the morning while Mom made beet pickles and did up a few jars of tomatoes. On the surface life looks normal but looks can be deceiving. I wonder what Dad is thinking about when he is alone in his shop working on something. Is he like me and when a task demands all my attention I can't think about anything else or does he constantly hear the words "I've got cancer, I've got cancer" whispering in his head. I remember when I was expecting the boys there wasn't a moment when I wasn't aware that I was pregnant. Just like there doesn't seem to be a moment when I'm not aware Dad has cancer. I just wish I knew what he is thinking. Is it constantly there? How could it not be? Does he have any peace or is he in a constant turmoil of emotions which he refuses to let us see?

Little by little, things are taking on a new "normal". Mom continues on with her domestic activities and devotes her time to caring for Dad and looks forward to spending time with the family. Dad is now fishing, making repairs to items, eating healthy meals and sleeping better. They have both returned to church and bake sales and are taking little walks around the village. And, like Mom, he is very interested in what individual family members are doing and looks forward to spending time with us. Life, while fraught with worry about Dad, is very good. We're happy (all things considered), healthy and still able to be together. For now, that's really all we should hope for. That's all we should ever hope for.

I can't say that I've done a lot of praying since all of this began. I just believe God knows what is in my heart. I believe He knows my fears and all the memories and emotions I'm experiencing. I guess I really just want strength or the promise of strength when I need it.

## Tuesday, August 30, 2005

*I'm* feeling a bit restless, like I'm in need of doing or experiencing something exciting. The trip to Ottawa just wet my appetite. I'd like to step away from the ordinary and do something unusual. I can't even say what it is I want/need to do. We've been extremely fortunate but I just need some little thing to add some sparkle. Wish I knew what!

# Part Four

# Autumn 2005

## Friday, September 2, 2005

*September!* Only a minute ago, or so it seems, I was listening to fireworks from a yard next to Gail's in Kingston to celebrate July 1st and the next I'm preparing to move out of the cottage on Labour Day Monday.

Ron left for Sharbot Lake early Wednesday afternoon so he was off the road long before it got dark. I've spoken to him everyday. Steve has told Ron he has officially earned his *Wood Pile'n License!* They've had a couple of really good, productive days. They've gotten all of Steve's wood brought down from the farm, they are going to do something with the pump from the lake at Mom and Dad's and they are going to cut a couple of logs at the farm for Dad. Then, this evening, they are going to the Perth fair to watch the demolition derby. Ron plans to leave for home early tomorrow morning. The house just isn't the same without him. Whatever would I do if something were to happen to him? He's such a huge part of me.

Gas prices rose to $1.295/liter this morning. Watching the news reports from the United States where Hurricane Katrina devastated Mississippi and New Orleans it's hard to believe it is the States the reporters are talking about. There are fears of disease such as Cholera and Malaria from the polluted water. The residents have no homes, no food or fresh water. The National Guard has been called in to take control of the streets. Looters are shooting people who try to protect their property. It's anarchy for sure! The oil rigs in the Gulf of Mexico stopped producing oil and no one knows how soon production will begin again. All of us may have to start walking more. Newfoundland is paying over $1.50/liter already. The economy will definitely take a beating.

Greg and I went to North Bay last night after dinner. I suppose, we should have stayed home and conserved the gas but old habits die hard and we really needed to do something different. I enjoy spending time with each of the boys. Greg has matured and we have a good time when we are relaxed and have time to hang out. We didn't buy much. Just ate dinner, went into a music store and looked around. Greg bought one disc. We picked up a few things Brandon might need to start school on Tuesday.

I don't feel as antsy today as I have been feeling. I have my accounts payables finished, the taxes sent out and things are in good order on my desk. Dad seems to be doing very well and when I know that I'm more at ease. I also know I'm going to spend some time with them next week and see first hand what a chemotherapy treatment is all about. I visited the high school today and got Greg out of a math class. He may have a small problem regarding his science class but a guidance councillor will help him next week. I also put Ron and me on a Bell Canada family phone plan so I can talk as much as I like to my family and pay only a minimal rate. So, I've accomplished a few things which have been weighing on my mind.

Something else has bothered me lately. When several of my friends were going through personal crisis I wrote them often and let them know I was there to support them without any strings attached. I guess that wasn't quite true. There was a string attached. I wanted to know they would support me when I experienced a bad time. These are people I thought for sure I'd hear something from but the silence has been deafening. I understand people sometimes don't know what to say, but a "Thinking of You" card usually says it all. I just don't understand and, stupidly, I'm hurt.

The sun is shining and the sky is brilliant blue so I'm hoping the weekend will stay that way. I'm looking forward to getting both Ron and Brandon home tomorrow. I miss my family when we are not together.

## September 6, 2005

*The* boys have returned to school this morning. Brandon seemed a bit nervous about starting grade seven at Land of Lakes Senior Public School, but wouldn't admit to it. Greg seemed relaxed and unconcerned about his first day of grade ten.

It has been a good summer. Not, perhaps, the summer we would have chosen but a good one none the less. Obviously, Dad's health has been at the front of everyone's mind but we were able to appreciate the time we spent together as a family and the adventures we've had.

Ron arrived home Saturday afternoon about 4:30pm. He said he and Steve had gotten lots of work done and had a good time besides. Mom and Dad were at Cathy's for dinner on Thursday evening and he and Steve helped do something with a pump on Friday. Friday evening Ron went with Cathy, Steve and Lindsay to the Perth Fair where there was a demolition derby. He said it was fun. Now, Dad is pleased that Steve's work has gotten caught up to-date and there shouldn't be any other work bees before winter. The next trip, as a family, will be the weekend of September 22 and we plan to play at the farm.

I'm heading to Sharbot Lake this afternoon. Dad's heavy chemotherapy treatment is tomorrow and then, on Friday, he has his appointment to determine what can be done about the tumor on his eye. Ron said it looked much better when he was there so perhaps the chemotherapy is shrinking the tumor. We can only hope. Dad's CT scan is scheduled for Saturday, September 17. This will indicate whether the chemotherapy is shrinking the other tumors and the results will also tell us how effective the treatment has been and if the cancer has spread anywhere else in Dad's body. This CT scan is very important not just for the physical aspect but also for our mental health. We need to know that he is going through all this and it is making a difference.

Brandon arrived home from hockey camp on Saturday afternoon. He had a great time and enjoyed staying at DJ's grandparents. Brandon's been away one week and I missed him so much.

We met the rest of Ron's family at his dad's house to celebrate Allie's 83rd birthday. Allie seemed to enjoy the attention and having us with him. Like Dad, Allie is very proud of his family and enjoys spending time with us.

Sunday was a great day. Ron brewed my coffee and while it was being made I went for a swim. The water was a bit chilly but not too bad. Then after our breakfast Ron and I took Casper for a walk. Later, Brandon came with us to a garage sale. We found a few pieces which we took back to our cottage. We hung out with the boys most of the day. Lauren and Derek came over in the afternoon to visit with the kids. The four kids watched a movie in the bunkhouse. It's the last night at the cottage. Lauren and Derek are heading home in the morning and we probably won't see them until next summer. I'll miss them. They are always zipping over on the sea-doo to visit with us. The summer has passed so quickly.

Monday morning dawned bright and sunny. I went for another swim. Ron and Casper came down to the dock to watch me. Then we stayed down there and talked and made plans for the day, for the week and for our future. The time Ron and I spend together at the cottage is the time I'll miss the most now that we are at home. We always seem to have places to go and schedules to follow. As hockey gets under way it gets even more intense and sometimes we barely have time to say Hi! I just love spending time with him. It's important that we find time to be together as a couple. That's one of the things I love about the cottage … it's our time.

We took Casper for a walk and then we began packing and cleaning. By 1pm we were ready to turn the lock on the cottage door and say good bye to summer. Ron says we'll spend some more time out at the cottage in September and to that end we left a few of the staples in the refrigerator so we have the basics when we do. There is some painting we need to finish and a few other little projects we'd like to do before the snow flies.

After we arrived back in the village we unpacked the vehicles and put everything away. We started a laundry and tidied the house. We all worked together and by the middle of the afternoon we had things in good order. The whole day has been a nice way to start the month.

I'm really not sure what to expect when I go to the cancer-treatment clinic tomorrow. I know the day will be long but that's OK if Dad is comfortable. I hate to be away the first day of school. I'd like to be here to listen to Brandon's tales of Land of Lakes Senior Public School, but I'll call this evening.

## Friday, September 9, 2005

*Today* is Greg's fifteenth birthday! Greg doesn't want to do anything to celebrate except meet his friends at the South River Fair. I got up early and decorated the dining area as per usual and he was allowed to open one of his gifts. He'll open the rest this evening.

The trip to Mom and Dad's and back home was very tiring. I arrived in Sharbot Lake shortly before six in the evening. Dad and Mom were in good spirits and were watching some of the game shows which are on TV in the evenings. After visiting and discussing the plan for the next day we all headed to bed around 9:10pm. I was tired so I really didn't mind an early night. The next day began at 6am and we left for Kingston at 6:45am. The day was long but quite interesting. Now, when they talk about the treatment, I'll be able to picture the room, the nurses and the process and that is very important to me.

Dad had his blood drawn at 8:15am and saw the doctor shortly before 10am. His weight went up by two pounds and his tumors which had been visible have shrunk. The doctor felt that was a very good indicator but I'm not willing to climb back onto the emotional roller coaster every time the doctor tells us something encouraging. It makes it so much more difficult when we're given bad news. His chemotherapy began at 11:05am and ended at 4:20pm. During that time we visited together and Mom and I went for lunch at the cafeteria in the hospital for a couple of hours.

Mom is very weary and has been living with this for so long. She is with Dad constantly, which I understand, but I feel she needs a bit of a break. I'm not sure what we can do to help her. A change of scenery for even a few hours might be helpful for her. We have been so focused on Dad's needs and the chores he would like to see done that we've, perhaps, overlooked Mom's needs. I don't want her to end up in the hospital from a stroke or exhaustion.

After Dad's chemotherapy was over we called Gail and Dad invited us out for dinner at the Chinese buffet in Kingston which they go to often. Seeing Gail was a real bonus which I hadn't planned on.

I drove home from Kingston which was cause for many jokes. Dad is a known back-seat driver and my driving in the city and then home had to have been hard for him. We arrived back in the village at 8:10pm. Yes, a very long day. We all headed to bed by 9:00pm to get a bit of rest. Dad was up a fair amount after midnight, and I heard him, but that is normal for the night of his chemotherapy. There are so many drugs in his system that he is wired for several hours. He sleeps quite a lot the next day.

Cathy came by for coffee on Thursday morning and I had a visit with her as well. Then around 11am I started for home. It was a good visit and I'm glad I went. I hope to be able to do it again before treatments end in November.

## Monday, September 12, 2005

*I* sent an e-mail to Mom and Dad's address by mistake on Friday afternoon. The e-mail was intended to be sent to Gail. The e-mail expressed concern for Mom and ways we could help her. She is very tired, almost a battle-fatigue tired, and, is alone with her thoughts whenever Dad is asleep. She is so amazing and we are all so proud of her but I'm also frightened this maybe too much for her. God knows it is almost too much for the rest of us. I can't imagine living under the constant stress of watching my husband slowly deteriorate without having some kind of physical reaction to it.

Mom and Dad were at an eye appointment in Kingston and I had to get Steve and Bradley to delete the message from Dad's computer. While the contents of the e-mail could have been read by

Mom and she would have understood, I was concerned Dad would see it. One of Dad's fears is being a burden on the family. His devotion to Mom is so complete he would have interpreted the e-mail to mean caring for him was hurting Mom's health. Therefore, it was imperative Dad not see the e-mail.

I called Cathy on Sunday and she was furious at me. Sending the e-mail to the wrong address was a careless mistake. I have been feeling awful about it since I sent the damn thing. My actions were not meant to be insensitive or cause any sort of a problem. Both Cathy and I said things we shouldn't have said to each other but I'm certain our confrontation was a release from the pent-up stress we each have been feeling. I'm sure Cathy feels the same.

I've read this type of conflict can happen with a prolonged illness. The family gets stressed and tired and eventually lashes out at each other as a way to vent. Emotions are high so arguments are inevitable. This journey will take us many places. A disagreement or two along the way isn't unusual. Our family's unity is very important to both Cathy and I and we'll recognize this for what it really is: frustration, anger and fear. There is nobody else we can yell at except each other. And we yell at each other because we know we are safe and we'll be forgiven. We'll be fine.

## Wednesday, September 14, 2005

*Today*, Dad is halfway through his 6-cycles of chemotherapy. Today's treatment is the short one and I hope things went well and they were able to get out of there without too much delay. I haven't heard from anyone except Dad yesterday or today. I know Gail is busy as she is Acting Boss at her office and will likely call tonight to tell me how things went.

## Saturday, September 17, 2005

*Dad* is scheduled to have his CT scan done today. Hopefully, the scan will show some positive results from the chemotherapy treatments. Dr. Gregg told Dad that he thinks Dad already knows the answer to whether or not the chemotherapy is working. I think that sort of an answer is very inappropriate. It gives us hope based on nothing more than the doctor's optimism. There are some positive signs. The tumor on Dad's eye has shrunk to half the size it was and the tumors on his head, side and back have also shrunk or disappeared completely. While I want desperately for the scan to reveal the chemotherapy is working I'm afraid to climb back onto the emotional rollercoaster only to have the doctor report to us something which is less than positive.

## Monday, September 26, 2005

*To* celebrate Dad being half through his 6-cycles of chemotherapy our family gathered at the farm in Arden for the weekend. We had a really wonderful time and the weather co-operated, as usual. Cathy and Mom had organized a turkey dinner for Saturday evening complete with all the trimmings. Gail ordered a fresh turkey from the butcher's and brought it out with them from Kingston. Cathy made the dressing and it was put into the oven to tease our taste buds all afternoon.

Gail and Rob arrived Saturday morning and Cathy's family stayed the night at their camp which is the next property to the farm. In the morning, Ron and I walked to the corner of Clark Rd and Brock Rd and back. We did the return trip in about forty minutes which is a good guide for me when I walk the *Canadian Imperial Bank of Commerce Run/Walk for the Cure* this Saturday. I think my sister-in-law, Dawn, and I can do the 5k in about an hour since the walk Ron and I took was 4.4k.

Dad took Brandon and Lindsay over to one of the pastures to have target-practice. Brandon is very good at hitting a moving target and Grandpa was very proud of how well both the kids did. Greg was tired and didn't have much interest in shooting the gun. Brandon and Rob continued target-practice with the pellet gun after dinner.

We came away from the weekend with many precious memories and the sense of family which is so vital to all of us. Unfortunately, I wasn't feeling well. We had, what seemed to be, a normal weekend and I was very happy about how everything played out.

*Brandon*

*The last time we stayed there Grandpa took my cousins, Lindsay and Brad, and my aunt's boyfriend, Rob, and me out behind the hen house to shoot some targets with the 22. I shot a few times but couldn't hit the bull's eye. Grandpa said I'd done good and bragged about me to my Mom. I asked Grandpa to show me how it was done and he replied, "I'm getting too old and I can't hold the gun straight," but when he shot he knocked the target right off the tree!*

*It's not the same without Grandpa and we barely ever go there now. The adults say we should sell it but that's the last thing I want to do.*

## Wednesday, September 28, 2005

**Dad** has his long chemotherapy treatment today. It is also the day when Dr. Gregg, the oncologist, will tell us what Dad's most recent CT scan had revealed about the tumor. Since Cathy began her new job last week at the Medical Center in Sharbot Lake Gail has arranged to go to Dad's treatment with them. Mom and Dad insisted that they could drive into Kingston by themselves and Gail feels maybe this small bit of independence is good for Dad's self-esteem. I agree and I'm also glad she will be with them for the doctor's appointment. It's nice to have a few people listening to what the doctor says so we don't get things confused. Gail told me in her e-mail Monday that she will call tonight to let me know how things went.

Both boys have begun hockey. Brandon will find out on Saturday at his first league game in Huntsville, Ontario that he has been made captain of his team this year. He'll be so excited since he feels he can't be captain because Ron is the coach. Brandon and a couple friends have been selected as players to be called up one level to the Bantam team to play when they are short players and when Brandon's schedule allows it. Brandon is very excited about this. Greg has begun his first year of Midget hockey and has been working out at the gym a few nights a week. He has one more night of tryouts but the general buzz is that he and Brody will fill two of the four spaces on the team. Both boys played with the Midgets last year when the team was short players due to injuries.

I have a hair appointment today at lunch time and a massage is scheduled for tomorrow after work. Saturday morning the central vacuum will be installed. Then, Saturday afternoon Brandon plays in Huntsville and we're not sure yet if Greg will have a hockey game over the weekend.

On Sunday, Dawn and I are doing the Canadian Imperial Bank of Commerce 5k Walk/Run. Sometime during the weekend Ron and I need to spend time at the cottage getting the docks in and closing up. Even though we had planned to spend a weekend at the cottage we suddenly find it is October so there is no point waiting to officially end the cottage season. Its already over!

Ron leaves next Friday morning for his annual moose-hunt. He has hunted with Steve Fox and several of Steve's friends for eight years. They don't have much luck but they do have a lot of fun. He is expected to be home the following Friday which will also be our 16<sup>th</sup> wedding anniversary.

I am struggling to avoid falling into my traditional autumn depression. The idea that the warm weather is all but behind us, the hockey schedules will soon take over our lives, we have no plans to get away this winter, as well as the ever-present realization that Dad has cancer all make it difficult to look positively into the next few months. A year ago tomorrow we confirmed our plans to travel to Panama. From that moment on I had something exciting to look forward to over the winter months. I love to travel. I love to have that something special to plan towards. I like being someone who is always doing something interesting and exciting.

## Thursday, September 29, 2005

*Gail* called last night to give me the results of the CT scan. The news wasn't as encouraging as we had hoped; nor as positive as Dr. Gregg had lead us to believe. The main tumor on the lung appears to have grown from 5 mm to 7 mm. Hardly the news we were expecting but the doctor did qualify the results with this possible explanation. Dad's CT scan which they are using as the baseline was taken three months before chemotherapy treatments started. During those three months the tumor may have grown from 5mm to 8 mm and then the chemotherapy shrunk the tumor back to 7mm. We really have no way of knowing how large it was on the day he began treatments. This upsets me. However, Gail and I do see positive results. Since beginning his treatments his appetite has improved, the secondary tumors on his eye, side and head have disappeared which tells us something is happening. The CT scan taken September 17 will now be the baseline to compare future CT scan results. Obviously, Dad and Mom were disappointed. Gail was careful to keep reiterating to them that we really don't know what size the tumor was at the beginning of the treatments so we shouldn't lose hope. Dad wants to continue the treatments and Dr Gregg is encouraging him to complete the cycle. Gail and I have both decided we are not going to climb into a hole of despair over this news. Our test results will come after the next scan. I said from the beginning that the doctor shouldn't have been so flippant when he made a comment about Dad knowing what the test results would reveal. That was setting us up for disappointment and we have had enough disappointment regarding Dad's cancer. We can't keep getting these encouraging, unfounded reports and then have the factual results squash us! It just isn't fair.

I found myself to be quite unemotional when Gail called to give me this latest piece of news. There was nothing. No tears, no fear, no disappointment. It is almost as if I've got novocain running through my veins when it comes to Dad's cancer. I've taken myself completely off the rollercoaster. I just can't do this over and over again. I'm more than willing to do anything and everything to help, bolster and encourage Dad and Mom but I want to be very matter of fact and clear when it comes to what the doctors are telling us. Life is precious and life is over only at the last moment and until that moment comes we will continue on in as normal a manner as possible.

Dad's long treatment was yesterday and they didn't get him started until 11:45am. Normally he should be done around 4:15 or 4:30

but yesterday he didn't finish until after 5pm. The nurses said there had been a mistake made when his appointment had been booked. Anyway, after his treatment his appetite was good and he, Mom and Gail went to the Chinese Buffet they enjoy. Gail said he ate several good-sized plates of salad, roast beef and Chinese food plus dessert. They drove home and called Gail's cell phone while she and I were talking. I was glad to hear they were home safe and sound.

Gail is taking them to his next treatment and then he has a week to rest. I think I'll plan to go with them on his next long treatment which will be mid-October. Ron will be back from moose hunting and it won't be a problem for me to get away during the week. Perhaps Ron will go down for his next treatment at the end of October. Now that Cathy is working fulltime she isn't able to get time off as easily. Dad's treatments, for this session, will end November 16, so I think Gail and I can handle it with some help from Ron. If he is scheduled for more treatments over the winter months we'll figure out our routine then.

Gail said Dad has been thinking about another trip and he can go if his condition doesn't change for three months after his treatment is finished. If he doesn't have more treatments he would be able to go the end of February. The sunshine and something positive to look forward to may be helpful as well. Since Cathy won't have time off perhaps Gail and I could consider traveling with them in case something was to happen while they were away. We'll see. As long as the weather was sunny and warm I don't think we would need to travel a huge distance. Get there and get settled. That would be the agenda for the first day. Anyway, I will wait to see what happens after he completes his 6th-cycle and whether the doctor feels another six cycles are recommended. If that happens, he wouldn't be able to travel until the summer

I e-mailed Dad and Mom this morning and I really didn't know quite what to say. Obviously, they know I was talking to Gail so I had to mention the scan results. I was factual and reiterated what the doctor had told them about the next test being a true indicator. I then went on to recount lots of little happenings from our life and I hoped what I had said was what he needed to hear. Results a bit more positive would have been a huge boost for both Dad and Mom. It would have made everything they are going through count for something.

### Friday, September 30, 2005

---

Subject: Re: Hi, Mom and Dad
Date:    2005 Sep 30—11:40
From:   Harold Clark
To:      Susan Arnold

Hi, Susan and all;

The storm is over and it's nice and bright today. It's a little cooler but they say it's going to warm up over the next few days. We can see the smile on Greg's face when he made the midget rep team … some proud, I'll bet!

I suppose it is time for meetings to start again. You have such a busy schedule.

You will be pleased to have your central vacuum installed. It should be a real asset.

So there's snow in North Bay; keep it there for the Northerner's. We don't need it yet!

Nothing else here so I'll scat.

Take care and say hi to everyone and we will catch up with you sometime over the weekend.

Love Mom and Dad

# Wednesday, October 5, 2005

---

Subject: Re: Good morning!
Date:    2005 Oct 04—14:50
From:   Harold Clark
To:      Susan Arnold

Hi, Susan

We're having another great day; it's supposed to be like this through Thursday.

Glad you're meeting went well. We agree, there is nobody like a church group to put on a good meal.

Brandon is certainly riding high in hockey this year!! He was pretty excited to learn he is captain. It's nice to have Greg's classes worked out and he'll do fine now that he knows what is going to take place and when.

It's another good day health wise. I'm doing some odds and sods; putting some things away for winter, etc.

We talked to Gail for a bit last night. She did not have any damage from the storm last Thursday and is getting along fine. She and Rob took in the chili fest and went boating on Sunday as it was so nice and calm on the lake.

We don't have any other news. Say Hi to all and have, what's left of it, a good day.

Love Mom and Dad

I can't believe it is now October. The months are flying by. It's been five months since we found out about Dad's cancer; five emotional, fearful and exhausting months. There never seems to be a break. Dad's cancer is seldom far from our thoughts. I've said it before but, although Dad has the tumor we all have the cancer. It's consuming.

Today is the end of Dad's fourth cycle of chemotherapy. Just two more cycles to go. Next week he can rest and begin the fifth long treatment on October 19. I'm planning to call Gail this evening to find out how things went.

There is reason for celebration as Dad has been enjoying several very good days recently. He and Mom attended the Church Supper and visited with many family and friends while they were there. The next day, a beautiful, warm autumn day, they attended church and then went to the farm where they travelled around, the two of them together, on the four-wheeler for hours. They didn't get home until after five o'clock. Even more out of routine was their choice for Sunday dinner … a pizza! They sounded like they had a wonderful time and Dad said he'd felt the best he's felt in three months. In his e-mail on Monday he mentioned, again, how well he was feeling and they were busy working outside in preparation for the cold weather. They are trying not to overdo but I know it must be hard when Dad is feeling so well.

Ron has also said I should head to Sharbot Lake anytime I want to. That seems to be a double edged sword. I love to be with Mom and Dad but being there just underscores Dad's illness. Beware the woman who knows not what she wants!

# Friday, October 7, 2005

---

Subject: Re: Good morning!
Date:    2005 Oct 07—11:20
From:   Harold Clark
To:      Susan Arnold

Hi, Susan

Well; there has been a definite change in the weather. It was raining this morning about 5:30 and has kept it up pretty much since. The temperature is not going above 14 C today so we will put a fire in the wood stove in the basement to keep the dampness away.

The hunting gang is all raring to go. Ron will be tired if he doesn't get some shut eye before tonight but there's security traveling together. Hope they have some luck again this year.

Looks like you have a full weekend ahead. We are not sure what we are doing. Lindsay's grade 12 graduation is tonight and she works Saturday and Sunday at the beer store. Bradley works both days at the grocery store but we're not sure of his schedule. Gail thought she would catch up with us sometime over the weekend. Whatever takes place will be fine. Mom has scalloped potatoes and ham on the menu. (I'm hungry already!!!).

Nothing else of news here so I'll toddle along. Take care. Wish Ron lots of luck and say Hi to the boys.

Love Mom and Dad

---

Today is the Friday of Thanksgiving Weekend. The months are zipping along and I have no idea where the past five months have gone.

Gail called on Wednesday evening to tell me how things went at the Cancer Clinic. Dad and Mom drove into Gail's and picked her up there. She then brought them to the hospital and waited for a while then Dad insisted she leave and they would call when they were ready to go home. She felt they appreciated the support but were comfortable enough with the process to look at it as a lot of waiting. She then suggested I come down the day after Dad's next long-session of chemotherapy so I can have a visit with them and he can be more relaxed. He tends to get a bit contemplative prior to his treatment. I think this is a good idea but I'll wait to see what they think. Dad seems to be feeling much better. The doctor suggested taking some Tylenol for arthritis because Dad's shoulder has been extremely sore since the surgery. The doctors have dismissed his pain by saying it was a by-product of the surgery but the surgery was over three months ago. An overextended shoulder injury would surely heal in three months when the shoulder is not being used much. Dr Gregg finally decided it may be a touch of arthritis which has settled into a weakened joint. The Tylenol seems to have alleviated the pain and has allowed Dad to sleep much better through the night which translates into more rest and better days.

Greg and I went to the gym last night. As I looked around the building I realized how much I actually do enjoy going there. I feel a sense of accomplishment when I complete a workout and I like spending the time with Greg doing something we have in common. The gym is so convenient and has been apart of my routine for several years.

Ron and Steve leave for the north and moose country tonight! They will be driving throughout the night and will arrive at the camp intime for breakfast. Steve couldn't leave any earlier because Lindsay graduated from grade twelve this evening.

On Saturday the boys and I are heading to Brandon's Pee Wee game at 5:30pm. I think we may go a bit early so I can make a stop to pick up a bedspread I saw in one of the stores. We'll stop for dinner after the game.

I don't plan to cook a turkey for Thanksgiving Sunday. We'll have our turkey next week when Ron is home to enjoy it with us.

If the weather is nice on Monday I'd like to put away some of the lawn furniture and ornaments from outside for another year.

Next year I should consider taking a few days vacation time off while Ron is moose-hunting. I would get a lot of stuff done and not feel like I'm rushed off my feet getting everyone where they have to be.

## Thursday, October 13, 2005

---

Subject: Re: Ron's home
Date:    2005 Oct 13—14:50
From:   Harold Clark
To:      Susan Arnold

Hi, Susan

Thanks for the update. Glad Ron is home and not too tired from it all. Just talked to Cathy and she had not heard anything more from the gang. I understand they are going to dress out the moose in Steve's barn where they will be dry as it's still raining and overcast. That's using their heads!

Nothing new here so I'll scoot. Take care and we will be
talking to you soon.

**Love Mom and Dad**

PS I'll call Cathy and tell her Steve and the boys made it as
far as South River by 10:30 this morning.


Gail called my office this morning. Apparently, Dad and Mom had
a really bad day yesterday. Dad's shoulder have been giving him
considerable pain and he has been taking more of the painkillers
and they, in turn, have upset his stomach. The cycle is vicious. He
was pale and not eating and extremely emotional. For Mom, I
believe she has really reached a low point. She is tired, worried and
scared. The day was bad enough that Cathy wanted to know if I
would consider coming down next Tuesday evening and staying
until the weekend. Dad has his long treatment on the Wednesday
and Cathy and Gail thought having me around would be nice to
help give Mom and Dad something else to think about. Naturally,
I'll be there.

It is hard to hear he is suffering so much today when, from all
accounts, he had a really good Thanksgiving. Gail and Lindsay
started the evening off with an impromptu lip sync of some country
music. Before long, Dad and Mom were on the floor dancing the
two-step. Then, when Dad tired of dancing he pulled out the
spoons and played for quite awhile. Rob was videoing the entire
event so I can see it at a later date. Gail even said Dad again discussed the possibility of a family trip in February. We were encouraged and happy that life seemed to have reached some semblance of
our previous normal. I, of all people, should realize that this disease
encourages hope and then snatches it away just as quickly. When

Allie was fighting his battle we all just held on for dear life since every day brought another revelation.

I believe part of what has upset me so much is the fact that I will never view Dad the way I have my entire life. Even if the cancer goes into remission I will still be thinking, "He looks thin, he looks tired, and he's not eating." I will always be searching for signs that indicate the cancer has returned. I find myself "putting on a happy face" whenever I'm talking to him. I don't want him to worry when my arthritis is flaring up. I don't tell him when work is unbearable. I don't confide in him the way I used to because I know there is so much he'd like to do to help but he just doesn't have the energy and that alone underscores the reason for his fatigue. I'd like to ask how we repair little things around the house. Those were always good conversation starters and we would ask questions and learn from what he would tell us. Now, I don't mention what I don't want him to worry about. I miss my friend.

## Tuesday, October 25, 2005

*I* just spoke to Mom on the phone. Dad was sleeping. It is only 8:40am. Dad has been experiencing considerable pain in his shoulder and has been taking painkillers to give him some measure of comfort. The trouble with the painkillers is they make him very drowsy. He sleeps a good amount of the day.

I went to Sharbot Lake last Tuesday afternoon and stayed until Saturday. Things are not good. The weather has been rainy and bleak, Dad's stomach has been upset and he is in pain although he does his best not to complain. Mom has reached the end of her rope and finds herself in tears when she is alone more often then not. She would never dream of letting Dad see her tears. Mom doesn't have the physical strength to help Dad in and out of the bathtub or up and down the stairs to their bedroom. Dad is worried about Mom. Dad suggested to Mom the other evening that he should go to a hospital or a nursing home so Mom would be spared the caring for him. Mom was very upset by this suggestion and told Dad they were partners and she will continue to do for him and be there for him as long as he needed her and not to talk about such things again. She reminded him that he had been there for her in 1993 when her rheumatoid arthritis first flared-up and she could barely get around the house. We are a family who has always stuck together and this will be no different. Dad hates to think that he will become a burden to any of us. Their genuine regard for each other is inspirational to a younger generation who coined the phrase the "Me Generation." Dad is willing to sacrifice his time at home in order to spare Mom. And Mom is willing to sacrifice nights of sleep, days of holding a plastic container for Dad to retch into before a meal and sore back muscles from steadying Dad as he grows physically weaker in-order to keep Dad where he loves to be … at home. They are amazing.

Throughout this journal I've commented so often about how strong Dad has been throughout this entire journey. Mom is just as strong. She is Dad's equal in everyway. Mom is very soft and gentle. She is shy and prefers not to be the centre of attention. She is intelligent and aware but most of all she is tough on the inside. She is determined and courageous. She continues on regardless of how scared she is of the future. We've always known this about Mom and watch with delight and awe as she would hold her ground with dignity or get a point across in the nicest way possible to someone who didn't want to listen! Margaret Thatcher, Britain's first female Prime Minister, was called "the Iron Butterfly." I believe Mom has earned that title, too. Her strength was developed at an early age. Her mother, my grandmother, died when Mom was just eighteen.

Her older siblings had married and left home and Mom remained with her father, bedridden and blind from rheumatoid arthritis, to care for him, her young brother and the house. Her older brother took care of the farm. This was at a time when homes were heated by wood-furnaces and baking was done in the cook-stove. When other girls her age were working in jobs and meeting new people and starting their own families, Mom was at home, making sure her invalid father was properly cared for. Her older sisters returned on the weekends to help and to do what they could to make life less dull, but the day to day responsibilities fell on the shoulders of a young-girl who wanted desperately to go to school. Her quiet ways, her giving-nature and her determination in the face of adversity has inspired my sisters and me for a very long time. And now, her tremendous inner fortitude is being tested again. And once again, she proves she's ready for the challenge.

Even though I had been raised in the small village of Sharbot Lake and knew first-hand of its ability to close-ranks and look after its own, I was not prepared for such an outpouring of community support, concern and caring. Clearly, Dad and Mom had touched many lives in their almost fifty years as residents here. Going to the Post Office or the store is difficult for Mom only because everyone she sees wants to know about Dad's condition. She returned from the store one day to tell Dad he had too many friends!! There is just no escaping, even for five minutes, her reality. There is no reprise from the ever-present cancer. We are very blessed to live where people care so deeply and that is one of the things that defines a small community; people care.

I become depressed in the autumn because winter is long and isolating but I have so much to look forward to. My husband and children are healthy and I can count on them to get me through this nightmare event. But, for Mom, Dad's illness is the ending of so much. I can't begin to understand everything she must be feeling and coping with privately. Living with this illness around the clock for months is just far more than any person can without having the strain wear down the body and soul. As I watch, amazed, I recognized how very brave both my parents are.

On Wednesday, we left at 7am for the cancer clinic in Kingston. Dad was not well and slept most of the drive. Today Dad saw Dr. Farnell. She works with Dr Gregg. She assessed the entire package of symptoms Dad has been experiencing. His weight is 153 pounds; down from the 178 pounds he weighed when he was first diagnosed with cancer. Dr. Farnell determined Dad was not well enough to continue the chemotherapy treatment this week although his blood work indicated no medical reason why he couldn't. The doctor left the room for a brief time before coming back to tell us she had conferred with Dr. Gregg and, together, they determined the chemotherapy was not working and was, in fact, making Dad sicker. So, they have discontinued the chemotherapy treatments permanently.

Dr. Farnell has scheduled some more scans because she believes the pain in his shoulder is being caused by a tumor under the shoulder girdle which is pushing the bone and causing it to protrude noticeably. The tumor on his head has returned and so has the one on his 10th rib on his right side. They have set up scans for his torso and head on October 31st with a follow-up appointment on November 9th. The plan, at present, will be to arrange radiation treatments to shrink the tumors which are causing the pain and give him some measure of comfort.

As the doctor is speaking I watch Dad and then Mom to see if they are hearing what I'm hearing. Did the doctor just say the chemotherapy wasn't working? Did she actually say the cancer has spread and radiation is for pain management only? There was silence in the examining room for a moment before the doctor sought to fill the silence with soothing, positive comments. Dad accepted her words in the same stoic way he's handled every other piece of news. I could see the deep thought which was taking place behind his bright-blue, intelligent eyes. Mom, too, remained calm and strong. I have always admired both of them so much but the way they handled this latest piece of news was beyond anything I had ever witnessed before. I am so proud to be their daughter. Their quiet dignity was so inspiring and it was their strength which helped me keep myself in control. Once again I felt like a spectator rather than a participant in the scene being played out in this tiny room. Dad thanked the doctor for her candor and her time and we retraced our steps back to the waiting room. I could see Dad's strength fading and knew he needed to rest before we began our return trip to Sharbot Lake.

Each stage of Dad's illness seems to end with a physical exclamation mark. There doesn't seem to be any blurring; there is no doubt or uncertainty about where we are in the journey. We have, once again, entered another stage of his cancer and each one seems scarier than the stage we just left. At the very beginning, the doctor who did the original test which confirmed Dad had lung cancer, had said it was extensive and the best we could hope for would be to keep him comfortable. The other doctors sort of built us up for a let down and it looks like the first doctor knew what she was talking about. She had estimated Dad could expect six months before the final stage. It will soon be six months since I was told about Dad's cancer.

We left the centre lost in our own thoughts and returned to Sharbot Lake. We discussed a bit of what the doctors had said but mostly we were silent. Dad slept off and on and Mom starred out the window at the passing landscape. I had called Gail at work to let her know what had happened. I also called Cathy at work after we returned from Kingston and had some lunch. Cathy has a bad cold and can't come to see Dad and is finding out how frustrating it can be to have only the phone and other people to relay information. She admitted she could understand how I have been feeling being so far away.

Thursday was bleak. I racked my brain to figure out what we could do to help Mom. Leaving Dad for any length of time isn't an option and, truthfully, none of us wanted to be anywhere else. Mom just keeps going. On Thursday she and Dad did make arrangements to have their car serviced on Monday at the dealership they had bought it from in Kingston. They arranged to have the furnace serviced on November 14. Dad called to renew their subscription for the mobile phone in the car. I stood at the kitchen window as they made their calls in the family-room. The moment was surreal. From the other room I could hear Dad making these arrangements for all the autumn duties which needed to be looked after, as if it were any other year. As he confirmed the expiration date on the phone subscription I couldn't help but wonder if he'd be alive in a year's time to see that date. Later, when I spoke to Gail she decided to take Friday off and would come to Sharbot Lake sometime during the day. I decided not to say anything to Mom and Dad in case her plans changed and she wasn't able to come until after work Friday.

Friday morning I came down the stairs resolved to bring some life back into this house. I turned the radio on and flipped on several lights. It may be daylight but we certainly needed a bit of light to brighten the rooms. Then, I asked Mom to show me how to bake bread and shape the loaves. At first, she was reluctant but reconsidered and seemed to enjoy her role as teacher. Suddenly, the morning was gone and the aroma of fresh baked bread filled the house. Just as we were finishing lunch Gail and Mattie, her cat, arrived at the backdoor which was a great surprise for Mom and Dad. Gail is blessed with a rare energy and any room she enters brightens instantly. Dad has that quality, as well. Maybe it is charisma or maybe it is their life-force shining from within and drawing the rest of us to them.

Gail had brought the ingredients for a spare-rib dinner which she and I put together later in the afternoon. Bradley arrived after school to cut the grass and Steve came to show Dad his pictures from the moose hunt. While Steve was there Gail, Mom and I went for a walk around the village. The exercise and fresh, crisp air was good for all of us, and especially for Mom. Her spirits seemed to have brightened considerably as the day progressed.

After Mom and Dad went to bed Gail and I sat up and discussed Dad's condition as well as what help Mom needed. We also talked about a few little things which could be done to make life easier for both Mom and Dad. By bedtime we had a few plans in our mind which we wanted to discuss with Cathy.

Gail and Mom turned off the water to the outside hose and put it away for the winter on Saturday morning while I was upstairs packing. Leaving was becoming more difficult and this time was the hardest but I was proud of myself because I had managed to control my emotions the entire weekend and dealt with what was practical and immediate instead of thinking about the emotional side of things. I did have to fight to control myself on Thursday when Dad insisted on discussing the farm and how he wanted us to handle the various land parcels which make up the farm. He also seemed to need validation that we understood he had always tried to treat the three of us the same way and had been there to support us and advice us without telling us what to do. I could certainly tell him, without hesitation, that he had done all of that and much, much more. Dad seemed reassured. They want to have a family meeting regarding business and are a bit afraid the meeting will be too emotional to get anything done. I suggested we could start with a small meeting with just the five of us. They felt that would be a good idea but didn't want Ron and Steve to feel excluded which wouldn't be the case and since both men have said on several occasions it might be easier with just my sisters and our parents.

I left at 11:45am. Dad was sitting in his rocking chair and as I hugged him he told me to be good and to call when I got home. Then, his beautiful blue eyes held mine for several seconds. I felt as though he was giving me strength and was silently reassuring me everything was going to be OK. The moment passed but it was a moment I'll never forget. All the emotions I had held in check since my arrival Tuesday came pouring out as the miles passed.

Gail invited Mom and Dad to come back into Kingston with her on Sunday morning. She reasoned they would spend a quiet day in town and then, since she was off on Monday, she would be able go with them to the car dealership on Monday morning. Mom and Dad agreed to her plan and they called me from Gail's on Sunday. I think it was a great idea on many fronts. The change of routine was good for both of them. On Monday they had the car winterized. They went back to Gail's for lunch and after Dad rested Gail drove them home to Sharbot Lake and stayed for dinner before returning to Kingston Monday evening.
Gail brought a fold-up cane for Dad and was going to find an appropriate time to give it to him. He is experiencing some balance problems and the cane seems like a good idea and could help Mom

steady Dad as he moves from one room to another but it could also be an emotional trigger. I haven't heard yet how this went. Gail had planned to call me last night but I had a late council meeting and haven't touched base with her yet. I sent an e-mail to her this morning and will likely hear back from her before the day is over.

## 4 pm

I heard from Gail earlier this afternoon. She was rushing off to a meeting but wanted me to know Dad, himself, had reopened the topic of a cane and when Gail showed him what she had purchased he seemed relieved. In short, he was using it. She also set up a 550-piece puzzle on the dining room table. Together Mom and Gail framed the outside and then, according to Gail, Mom became inspired and was working away on it and was talking to Cathy on the phone at the same time. Hopefully, this will help to fill some of the dismal hours when it is raining outside and Dad is sleeping inside.

A week ago, at this time, I was heading my vehicle in the direction of Sharbot Lake. I've said it many times but, given the nature of Dad's illness, the speed in which time passes is of great concern.

## Friday, October 28, 2005

*Dad* e-mailed me this morning after I had sent a short note telling him what we are up to today and also telling him about the mother bear which had been shot within the town limits leaving behind three cubs. I could tell by his e-mail he was much worse.

---

Subject: Re: Good morning!
Date:    2005 Oct 28—10:54

**From:  Harold Clark**
**To:     Susan Arnold**
**Hi Susan Well!!! Geet (Sic) your gun Winter may be longer than you think. Don't think I want one of those on my back., (Sic) Nothing new hear so wll (Sic) scram Have a good day**

**Love Momand (Sic) dad.**

I took yesterday off. My entire system seems off. I'm nauseous and can't seem to find any food in the house which I find appealing. The mere thought of eating is almost repulsive. I think all I ate yesterday was a granola bar, a couple slices of toast and a dish of chicken soup. I really don't feel any better today and can't decide whether it is a flu bug or stress related.

I feel like I'm wasting what days God has given to me. There needs to be laughter and joy in life and surprises and anticipation and adventures and colour. Instead, I feel like there is just nothingness stretching ahead of me. Is this a normal part of my family's journey? Does the landscape look like this to everyone who must travel this road? We've never been here before.

Dad has been experiencing more pain and, as a result, is awake during the night because the pain is so hard to ignore. Losing Dad will be so very difficult but watching him suffer is so much worse. It breaks my heart to know I can't do anything to help him. I almost feel like Dad is already gone. Each time I see him he is a little thinner and a little shakier on his feet. He sleeps more often now and doesn't have the same interest in the topics we always used to discuss. He is, however, determined to beat the cancer and continues to make plans for the future. He plans to go deer-hunting the first week of November. Ron has said he will go to hunt with the guys if Dad goes and Mom feels quite secure knowing Steve, Cathy and Ron will all be there watching out for him. Ron will also take them to Kingston for Dad's appointment on the Wednesday and hear what the doctors have to say after his scans which will be taken this Monday (the 31$^{st}$). Cathy is going to be with them for the scans. Hopefully, these scans will give us a better indication about what we are dealing with. I see Dad failing and need to make some plans for spending time with Mom and Dad.

I called Mom and Dad around 1pm this afternoon. Dad had eaten his lunch and was sleeping. Mom says he's so weak she practically has to lift him out of bed and, when it is nighttime she has to help him to bed. During the day he wakes up long enough to take his pills and then goes back to sleep. Personally, I feel the painkillers are too strong for him since they have codeine in them. I suggested Mom ask Cathy to arrange with the pharmacist in Sharbot Lake to have the prescription for Tylenol 3 be transferred to Sharbot Lake from the hospital pharmacy in Kingston. He would then have the pain medicine without the drowsiness and getting the medicine would be more convenient.

Mom said they had a busy day yesterday. Several visitors stopped in for a visit later in the afternoon. The Eastern Star had a luncheon today at the church and an uncle of mine brought a tray of soup and sandwiches over to their house. In normal circumstances Mom and Dad would have supported the event by attending. Everyone is so thoughtful. The smallest gestures bring the greatest comfort at times like these.

I asked Mom if she was finding a way to fill her time while Dad slept. She sounded better than she had last week and assured me she was keeping the radio on for company and was also working on the puzzle she and Gail started last week. She said she didn't do too much housework aside from laundry and meals but I told her not to worry about anything else so she didn't get more tired out. The fact that so many people were in during the past couple of days would do her as much good as it does Dad. Maybe more.

I think the next time I visit Sharbot Lake I will plan to attend church on Sunday. I'm usually packing up to leave at the same time the service is on. I feel the need to visit the church a few times before I'm there for another purpose. That church has a long history with our entire family. Many of the people who used to attend are no longer there but I still feel at home there. I'm starting to feel the pull towards my religious roots.

## Monday, October 31, 2005

*Dad's* health is in rapid decline.

Mom called Gail on Friday and asked her to pick up the Tylenol 3s. Gail said she'd bring them to Sharbot Lake on Saturday. I knew Gail hadn't planned to go to Sharbot Lake this Saturday so when I heard she'd been to Mom and Dad's I knew instinctively that something wasn't quite right.

I was antsy all day Saturday. Part of me wanted to call and yet the other part of me knew I'd fall to pieces.

On Sunday Mom called me. She was putting on a good front but from the onset of the conversation I knew things had changed. Mom told me Cathy was in the family room with Dad and she was clipping his fingernails. Steve had gone up to the farm to trim a path for Dad's truck so he wouldn't have to walk during hunting season.

Mom told me Rob and Gail had been out and had brought enough food to feed an army but couldn't stay to eat any themselves. Warning bells went off in my head.

Cathy picked up the extension in the family-room and asked me when I was coming back to Sharbot Lake. Although she sounded calm there was something in her tone of voice. She didn't talk for long. I asked Mom if Dad was sleeping or if I could speak to him for a minute. She hesitated, but Dad took the phone. He barely spoke and when he did I couldn't make out much of what he said. I chatted on about what the boys were doing and told him a few things I was up to. It was obvious talking was tiring for him and he asked me if I wanted to speak to Cathy. I said I would. Before he hung up he said, "Be good". I had been on the edge emotionally for the entire phone call but had remained calm and in control until he said those words which rang out loud and clear. They were so normal sounding in an abnormal conversation.

I couldn't speak to Cathy through the constricted throat and the tears. She told me they'd call later. When we hung up I dissolved into tears at the kitchen table. Brandon was in the living room and Greg was downstairs. Ron had taken Casper for a walk and it was because of his absence I hadn't phoned Mom and Dad's. I was waiting for him to be with me.

I went for a shower to wash away the tears. When I was finished it was evident the boys had filled Ron in on what had happened when he and Casper had returned. Ron was sitting downstairs alone when I found him. I tried to pretend I was fine but the tears began all over again. He put his arms around me and let me sob. I cried so hard I ended up making myself sick. I was a mess. I sat next to the toilet in the laundry room and cried until I couldn't cry any more. Ron was ready with his arms when I came out. He decided we would drive out to the cottage and take a few things back that we had brought in from the lake by mistake. The drive would give me a chance to think and adjust to another stage of this damn disease.

The drive gave me time to gain my composure and the blue skies and colourful autumn grasses and leaves couldn't help but lift my spirits. The rest of the day alternated between tears and chores. Ron and I packed away the seasonal clothes and clothes slated for disposal were put into garbage bags. Allie wasn't feeling up to dinner but Ron took him down a plate. I had made mashed potatoes, Swiss steak with gravy and peas. I didn't eat much. I couldn't. My stomach has been unsettled since Thursday.

After dinner Steve called. He said things weren't good. Dad had failed visibly since I saw him a week ago. Steve told me he wasn't telling me what to do but I should spend my time in Sharbot Lake. The raw emotion in Steve's voice and the words he wouldn't say made it very evident Dad's cancer seemed to be winning the battle. I called to Ron. He and Steve spoke for awhile and made plans for us to go down and then Cathy wanted to talk to me. Cathy had spent Friday night at Mom and Dad's. He is far too weak for Mom to help up and down the stairs. The pain is bad and he requires painkillers but they don't seem to be helping. Mom has agreed to have some apparatus delivered this morning. Cathy ordered a chair with a spring seat for the family room, a commode chair for downstairs and a higher toilet seat for upstairs. A bath seat which requires Dad to sit on it and then turn into the tub is also arriving. Mom put the wall up when Cathy mentioned a hospital bed. I can understand why she couldn't permit the bed to arrive just yet. Mom knows Dad isn't getting better. The other tools are helpful implements but moving Dad into his own bed brings death so much closer. So,

Cathy didn't push. The time will come and Mom will make the decision. Dad is disoriented and seems quite confused at times. He is sick to his stomach more often; even with the anti-sickness pills he has been taking. Dad and Mom had stayed in Kingston at Gail's house last Sunday and Monday. Gail arrived in Sharbot Lake on Saturday and was shocked by how much Dad had failed in five days. Steve told me I'll be shocked. Unless things change we are planning to arrive in Sharbot Lake on Sunday. The plan is for us to drive Mom and Dad to Kingston as he has an appointment for his scans at 11am on Monday morning. However, plans change. Dad has an appointment, a radiation consult, today at 2pm and Cathy has arranged her schedule to be with them. She will let Gail know how the appointment goes and Gail and I will be in touch.

I said to Ron I think I'm still in shock even after all this time. Even after all my tears. I just can't really believe this has happened to our family. Even more, I can't believe we can't do anything to change the outcome. I'm not really sure if Greg and Brandon really understand what is happening. They know Dad has cancer but so did Allie. Allie had cancer twice. I'm so afraid they are in denial; especially Brandon. I'm also afraid I can't help them. I know I should because they are my children and I never want them to be hurt but I'm in more pain then I've ever been in my entire life. I'm not just losing my Dad but I'm losing my oldest friend. He has been with me every step of the way. Always teaching, advising, teasing, supporting, challenging, encouraging, discussing and sharing the little moments in my life as well as the larger ones. In looking back upon my life I realize the little moments were the important ones and they are why I am finding this latest challenge so difficult. Parents are supposed to leave us and pass into eternity but friends are supposed to stay and share the joys and tears. Dad is supposed to hear about the boys' and their hockey. He's supposed to settle into a lawn chair or lounger and tell a joke or cause some mischief. He valued the simpler things in life because he knows they are the important things.

At the end of my work day Ron's cousin, who works for us at our store, came into the municipal office. She asked to speak to me. Steve Fox had been trying to reach Ron and I. Ron wasn't at the store and the home phone was busy. Steve had told Karen to find me and phone his cell phone. Dad had been admitted to the hospital in very grave condition. The calcium levels in his blood stream where very high which means his bones were starting to break down. The calcium causes nausea and disorientation. He was also very dehydrated and the doctors give him only a couple of weeks to live. The end was approaching quickly. I began to shake and cry and the confusion in my brain was no less then the reaction from an unexpected trauma. I had thought about this moment many times but the reality of it still isn't sinking in. Patty put her arms around me and Karen put my coat on me and said she'd drive me home. I regained what few wits I still owned and said I was fine to drive home. Karen tried our home number again to tell Ron what was happening. She followed me home to make sure I got there in one piece. I had told Steve to call us again in half an hour. Ron spoke to him and I had a total melt down in our bedroom. I didn't want the boys to see me in this condition. They were aware of what was happening but I just couldn't let them see me in such a state. I'd like to think it was my maternal instinct protecting the boys from seeing me so distraught but I suspect there was also a bit of pride keeping me away from the boys. Ron stayed with me in our room to help me calm down, he brought me a glass of water and as I began to make sense of this latest development we began to discuss the practical side of our heading to be with the family. We had to leave for Kingston the next morning. Dad was stable for the moment and wasn't in any immediate danger. Ron dished out the candy to the spooks and goblins and I returned to the municipal office where I put the finishing touches on a few things which needed to be done since I didn't know when I'd return. After arriving back home I packed and all of us headed to bed to get whatever sleep we could.

## Tuesday, November 1, 2005

We arrived at the hospital in Kingston around 3pm. Dad was doing OK but was very sleepy. We went into his room to see him and he looked so pale and small in the hospital bed. I was able to kiss him on the forehead and he woke up long enough to say Hi. We stayed at the hospital and took turns sitting with Dad until visiting hours were over. We found it difficult to leave Dad while we headed home to Sharbot Lake. Gail had decided to stay a little while longer. I drove Mom home in their car and Ron followed with our car and the boys.

## Wednesday, November 2, 2005

We found Dad looking so much better when we arrived at the hospital this morning. Gail was already there and said he'd had a pretty good night. Gail had actually stayed the night with Dad because he was so disoriented and the floor nurses didn't seem to have much time to look after all the patients. In fact, the nurse who came on duty at 11 o'clock didn't check on Dad until 2:30am and that's when she discovered Gail. The nurse wanted Gail to leave immediately but Gail was determined to stay. Gail told her she'd received permission from the nurse in charge on the previous shift and, since her car was parked in the underground parking lot, she'd be staying where she was until the morning. Gail also observed the time was 2:30am and the nurse was just then finding her and that meant she hadn't made her rounds after coming on the floor. It was decided Gail could stay!

The room was the only bed they could find for Dad when he was admitted and soon after lunch he was moved to the cancer palliative floor. The staff, there, were more compassionate. Cathy knew some of them. By the evening Dad had perked up quite a bit and, while the family was all around him and a couple of the grandchildren were sitting on his bed, Dad enjoyed a beer the doctor had told him he could have. He was in good spirits and visited and joked with everyone. Aside from the hospital setting it was like any other time we get together. We were joking and poking fun at each other and Dad was chatting with everyone. Mom sat in the chair next to Dad's bed and held his hand. I'm glad my boys could see him like this. They are leaving tomorrow and whether they know it or not this will be their last visit with Grandpa. Ron, Mom and I have discussed this from many angles and we feel this is best. I want them to remember all the good times and not his deathbed.

## Thursday, November 3, 2005

*This* morning Mom and I drove her car to the hospital in Kingston and Ron and the boys drove behind us. They are leaving this afternoon for South River and Mom and I are staying in Kingston at Gail's. Mom seems focused and resigned to where this is heading and I don't seem to be having a lot of emotional waves, either. I guess we're just dealing. Mom needs me and I need her and that makes it easier to concentrate on the moment.

Dad is still moving a fair amount. He will sit up with his legs over the side of the bed to eat his meals. I usually put a pillow the long side against his body and then I sit with my back to him to make a back rest while he eats. We think it works fine. He still gets up and, with assistance, walks to the bathroom. Even a little bit of exercise seems to tire him out. The nurses don't seem to be able to get into see him and when he needs to be taken to the bathroom or moved in his bed we end up doing it but then we're told not to because we're not covered by hospital insurance if we hurt our backs. Too damn bad! If Dad needs something and the nurses can't help him then we sure aren't going to let him stay very long in one position or let him wet the bed. They have been over medicating him. Dad would only ever take half a Tylenol when he had a headache and the doctors have prescribed two Tylenol #3s every four hours. This would keep him unconscious if we hadn't asked them to lower the dosage. The nurses are pleasant enough but I think they would prefer it if we weren't around so much. If his medication keeps him sleeping then they have less to do for him. The floor is crowded and the nurses are few so I can understand how they might feel but I don't want my father to be kept in a comatose state to make things easier. This is about making Dad's quality of life the best it can be for the time we have left. Just as other families struggle to do the same thing for other patients.

When it came time for Ron and the boys to leave I could feel my emotions starting to swell. My chest hurt, my throat ached and my eyes were stinging from unshed tears. First Greg gave Grandpa a hug and then Brandon did. Grandpa told them to be good boys and good luck with their hockey on the weekend. I had to step out into the hall. Dad told Ron to be careful and Ron told Dad he'd see him on Sunday. I can't even explain the emotions I was feeling. Everything is happening so very fast.

The days are long at the hospital. Nobody is feeling very hungry and the hours just seem to go on and on. It is so strange to be with Dad and not be visiting and asking him questions. Only the moment we are in seems to matter. Only his creature comforts and how he's feeling seems important. The magazines we try to read remain opened at the same page and each time we start to read the article it is as though we had never seen it before.

Gail, Mom and I went home to Gail's place when visiting hours ended. At least Mom and I will have a break from traveling that dark highway home to Sharbot Lake.

*Brandon*

*Going to see Grandpa at the hospital was the hardest thing I had done and probably ever will do. Grandpa was always so strong and independent and now he couldn't even get out of bed. He looked so weak and sick but he still found a way to always be smiling at me.*

*The first day we spent at the hospital was boring but I knew it was worth it. Grandpa was sick and sleeping most of the time. I had a cold so I had to keep my distance from Grandpa and wear a mask when I wanted to get closer. Everybody was really worried and tired but nobody wanted to go home. My brother and I stayed for two days and then Dad took us back to South River.*

*The night before we left Grandpa was feeling better and we managed to sneak him in half a beer. We all sat around his bed and I was even on it with him and we told jokes and talked. It was great!*

*The next day we went straight to the hospital to have a visit before we left for South River. He wasn't doing so well anymore. We didn't have much time with him before we left. My brother and I each hugged him and he said, "Be good boys, now" and then we left.*

*I knew that was the last time I would ever get the chance to talk to him again. I know it sounds babyish but I cried half the way home. Mom stayed at the hospital with Grandpa and Grandma.*

*The doctors told Grandpa there was nothing more they could do to help him so he asked if he could go home.*

*Dad brought us home and got us organized and then he went back to be with Mom and the rest of the family. I was glad Dad brought us home; I didn't want to see Grandpa any worse than he already was.*

*From that day on I haven't any desire to do my work or anything. I just want to build a time machine and go back to when my Grandpa would put on his Santa hat and pass out gifts. I knew that wasn't going to happen so nothing even mattered any more.*

### Friday, November 4, 2005

*We* found Dad in good spirits when we arrived at the door to his room in the morning. Dad seemed to have slept well last night and had eaten breakfast, was washed, shaved and was sitting up waiting to greet us.

As always, his first questions were about the family. How did Mom sleep? How were we? Did I hear from Ron and the boys last night? What time did they get home to South River?

A few days earlier Gail had brought Dad her digital clock which told the day, the date and the temperature as well as the time. The digits were large and easy to read from a distance and Dad used it to help keep him oriented. He slept quite a bit during the day and found he was getting confused about what day it was. The first thing he would do each time he woke-up, day or night, was consult the clock.

I had brought him a few little incidentals for his comfort. The hospital air is very dry so I brought him a nose gel to keep the inside of his nose moist. His lips were dry, too, but the waxy balms seem to feel worse to him then the cracked skin. We would keep his arms, legs, hands and feet creamed with a body lotion and he liked the feel of his housecoat over his pajamas.

He didn't seem interested in reading the newspaper or having it read to him. That was a significant change. Always, Dad was interested in what was going on in the outside world. We are also discovering his need for us to slow down our sentences and our movements. Gail asked him several questions, one after the other at a normal, conversational pace. His brain couldn't comprehend as quickly as she could ask the questions. If we moved around his bed too much the motion seemed to bother him.

He has had several visitors everyday. Dad and Mom's minister has been in to say Hi quite often the last few days. When the visitors had gone Dad would either slip off to sleep or talked quietly to Mom. Gail and I would leave them alone to give them their private moments and we would head down to the family room and either chat about Dad's condition or we'd both stare at a television which was turned on in the corner of the room. We quickly developed a routine and the hospital rooms and the staff in the halls became as familiar to us as our own families and our homes. We learned which toaster in the tiny kitchenette burned the bread and which cupboard held the tea and sugar. We marked the passage of time with the sound of the shaky, metal carts carrying the lunch and dinner trays as they drew closer and closer to Dad's room.

Cathy and Steve and the kids would come to the hospital after work everyday to visit and then we'd leave when the nurse came to get Dad ready for the night. We'd all kiss him good night and tell him to get some rest. He'd tell us to be careful going home and to get a good nights' sleep, too. Then, like clockwork, he'd always tell us not to come into the hospital so early. We should stay home and rest. And, like clockwork, we'd assure him we were fine and we'd see him in the morning.

## Sunday, November 6, 2005

---

Subject: Attention Patty/Raina
Date:    2005 Nov 6—21:47
From:    Susan Arnold
To:      Village of South River

Hi, Girls, Happy Monday!

Just a note to tell you Ron and I are planning to return to South River tomorrow for a day or two. Dad has been stabilized for the time being. He is lucid enough to know I am away from the boys and the office and is beginning to fret over this, so, if things are still well tomorrow we will be home in the evening. I plan to be in the office on Tuesday and part of Wednesday so perhaps, Patty, we can plan to sit down together to go over anything and everything you will need to know. At that time I will make a formal request to be absent from work. We hope to be able to bring Dad home although we know it will be a challenge but it is what everyone wants. You know us, we make decisions as a team and this was no exception. The doctors felt when he was admitted on Monday that his condition was very grave but he rallied. He will continue to decline from here on and it will really be up to Dad how long he wants to fight. It could be a week or it could be a month. Anyway, I can't seem to concentrate completely on things here because I feel as though I left you so suddenly and need to return to help you get familiar with everything. Could you please have any questions, concerns, invoices, messages, etc listed for me and we'll go through them together on Tuesday. I really miss seeing both of you and hearing about your lives.

Enough mush! I'll bring the coffee and you bring the fun and we'll get everything sorted out. If anything changes and we won't be returning tomorrow I'll try to get in touch with you either directly or indirectly.

Surprisingly, we're all doing really well. Hope you are too.

Looking forward to being home and seeing you.

Susan

## Monday, November 7, 2005

*Dad* is sleeping so much. We try to get to the hospital early enough in the morning to see the doctor when he makes his rounds. We want the doctor to reduce Dad's medication because he isn't in significant pain and the medication makes him so sleepy. A regular dose has always been too strong for Dad. Fortunately, today, we arrive in Dad's room just ahead of the doctor. Dad is still sleeping when we make our request. We are able to speak knowledgably to the doctor which, I think, goes a long way in having him make the decision, based on what we've told him, to reduce his medication. We know what time Dad has been given his pills and when he is due for more. Dad doesn't like being asleep so much of the time. He wants to be awake and aware of his surroundings.

Even though everything is marked on Dad's chart our family is keeping our own chart in a small notebook. We would never have it where the nurses could see it to make them feel we didn't trust them but we feel it was appropriate to, as a carpenter might say, "measure twice and cut once". Mistakes, unfortunately, can and do happen and it doesn't hurt to ask questions when a pill is a different color or a different form from how it is normally administered. This journal was our way of double checking Dad's progress. We wrote down when he ate, what he ate, when he went to the bathroom, when he had his medication and how long he slept. And; it gave us something to do which, we felt, was useful.

There is real time and there is hospital time. In the hospital there is only now and our existence becomes almost cocoon-like. We don't fear the future because it just doesn't exist. Only what is being said or done at this very moment is important. Little things take on a new meaning. Eating his entire pudding cup seemed to mean Dad's appetite was improving. Having him catch us with a small play-on-words would mean he was feeling better. Dad can never miss an opportunity to play a joke, even a small one! Just seeing his blue eyes sparkle with mischief was like a gift from Heaven!

Ron and I are returning to South River this evening. I feel as though I left the office in such a hurry and there are things I really need to complete before I can concentrate completely on Dad. I miss the boys and I want to spend sometime with them. We'll come back on Thursday, prepared to stay as long as Dad and Mom need us to stay.

Dad seems to be stable and is starting to become a bit agitated because he knows I'm taking time off work and I'm not with the boys. He has never been comfortable being the centre of attention and he has never wanted to inconvenience anyone on his behalf. Doesn't he know we'd rather be with him? I asked him before his surgery in June when he was saying don't come down, "Where would you be if the roles were reversed?" We didn't need to discuss it again. He would be right beside each one of us all the way. He'll be content knowing we're going home to look after our responsibilities even if it is only for a few days.

## Tuesday, November 8, 2005

*Today* is Mom's birthday. I called her this morning to tell her I was thinking about her. "Happy Birthday" just didn't seem appropriate. She sounds tired on the phone. I wish, with all my heart, I could do something to help her. She is such a gentle woman but has always had the strength of spirit which allows her to keep going and helps her do what she has to do. As she says, "What else can I do except go on?"

It was nice being back at the office but it felt a little strange, too. Everything was so normal and I feel as though I've been in a totally different world. I suppose, I have been. The distraction at the office was good.

I have missed the boys so much. I just want to sit and hug them for hours. Naturally, they aren't prepared to do that for me! They have really stepped-up to the plate and are handling life here without us so well. I'm so very proud of both of them.

Uncle Steve Arnold comes at night to stay with them and to make sure they get the bus for school in the mornings. Greg does the laundry for both of them and Brandon has made several of their meals. He is a grilled-cheese king! The family has invited them for meals and we left groceries for them. All in all, they are doing fine.

We call them every day at least once and most days it is twice a day. I like to feel we're still apart of their lives.

## Wednesday, November 9, 2005

*Ron* and I have returned to Kingston. The doctor has told the family the cancer is now in Dad's organs, his brain and his bones. Dad was awake when the doctor came to see him. The doctor, Dad and Mom talked about what the next step should be. The cancer team has determined they are going to give Dad radiation on the shoulder to give him some relief from the terrible pain the tumor is causing under the shoulder girdle. The radiation is only to keep him comfortable; the outcome would not change. The treatment is scheduled for Thursday. The process was explained to Dad and Mom. Then Dad was asked if he wanted to remain in the hospital or if he'd like to go home.

"I'd like to go home and be with my family."

Plans are now being made to have hospital equipment and oxygen delivered to Mom and Dad's house for Friday. The paperwork is being done to get Dad on the Home Care Nurses patient list.

I'm really not sure how much breakfast Dad is eating in the mornings. This is the only meal we aren't present for and judging from how poor his appetite is the rest of the day I can't believe he is eating as much as he says he is. Maybe he is confused and is listing the food that was on the breakfast tray. Or, perhaps, he's thinking we won't worry so much if we thought he was eating something. Or, perhaps, his confusion makes him believe he did eat breakfast.

One nurse, who was talking to us about caring for Dad at home, told us the loss of appetite is normal at this stage. The key is keeping him hydrated and even his thirst sensation will disappear. She reminded us to keep a sheet underneath Dad which will enable two people to grasp the four corners and shift him up in the bed when gravity has caused him to slip down. The sheet makes it more comfortable for the patient and helps prevent injuries from lifting incorrectly. She also advised us to make sure we take care of our own needs: we must get proper food into our system and not rely on "fast food" and coffee to sustain our bodies. We must keep ourselves hydrated and take a few minutes everyday and go off by ourselves. Alone time is at a premium but so necessary for care-givers to allow energy to be recharged and emotions to be dealt with. And, she encouraged us to get some fresh air everyday. Her advice was sound and practical and derived from many years of experience. She didn't diminish how hard it will be caring for Dad at home but spoke about what a truly wonderful gift this time together will be for our whole family. Dad should be surrounded by the people and the things which he loves. If we can do this for him I feel we will have done everything possible to help Dad through this final part of his journey.

A physiotherapist came into see Dad this afternoon. She was insistent that Dad needed to get up on his legs and get them moving. She brought him in a walker with large rubber wheels and a seat on it in case he needed to rest. Dad agreed, more to get her to leave him alone then for any other reason. He took hold of the walker and took off down the hospital hall so quickly the therapist had to run to keep up with him! His head was held high in the air and I could see the "I'll show you" body language he was displaying. Now *that* is my Dad! Just give him a challenge and then get him a little annoyed! Part of me wanted to laugh because it was something I had seen so many times and the other part of me wanted to cry to see him heading down the hall with the walker. Dad has always had a quick walk with a purposeful step. He had a straight-up-the-back posture which set him apart from those around him.

Mom reached over to take my hand but her eyes never left Dad as she watched him pushing the walker down the hall.

### Friday, November 11, 2005

*Ron* and Gail brought Dad home today. Mom and I stayed in Sharbot Lake to take delivery of the hospital bed and the oxygen. The livingroom resembles a hospital room but at least Dad will be home with us. Remembrance Day will always have another memory attached to it for our family.

The doctor had already been around to visit Dad, had discharged him and had ordered the medications which were to accompany Dad home. Gail went to the hospital pharmacy to wait for the prescriptions to be filled. Dad was more than ready to leave the hospital and the longer he had to wait the more impatient he grew. He had not wanted to be brought home in an ambulance. He had elected to arrive in his own vehicle which wouldn't draw as much attention on a busy Friday morning in the Village of Sharbot Lake.

The trip home exhausted him and he practically collapsed on the bed when we got him inside. In the past two days his leg muscles have lost most of their strength and he required two of us to help him into the house. He was sore and didn't want to be jostled around once he was on the bed. He slept soundly for most of the day.

With Dad now home with us we felt, for a bit, like new parents who suddenly find themselves responsible for their tiny charge. Suddenly, we were responsible for Dad's care and comfort and the task ahead of us looked very daunting. So, we did what we usually do; we sat down to make a plan.

Cathy was still working through the day but she was able to drop by at lunchtime to see Dad and then she would return in the evening to help prepare him for the night. Gail, Ron and I were going to be staying with Mom and Dad so we began discussing what our routine needed to include.

We set up a little table next to Dad's bed and stocked it with tissue, body lotion, his spit up dish, a glass with water for Dad to sip on a regular basis and the baby monitor base. We could move the intercom part around the house so we could hear when Dad was awake or needed help. In the kitchen we kept a pitcher of ice water in the refrigerator, purchased some flexible straws and bought some pudding cups and gelatin which Dad had eaten in the hospital.

We began to sort through the medications the hospital had sent home with Dad. Each of us, at first glance, had commented on the number of different drugs that had been sent for Dad. He hadn't taken this many drugs when he had been hospitalized. We checked all the labels and they were, indeed, prescribed for Harold Clark. We began sorting by the medications we knew Dad had been taking. We found the painkillers, the drug which kept the brain from swelling, the anti-nausea pill, the stool softener and then we discovered a laxative, a heart pill, an antihistamine and something else we weren't familiar with. Something was wrong. These drugs couldn't be for Dad. He didn't have a heart problem and not once had the doctors indicated one could develop during these last few weeks. The laxative would cause tremendous stress on a body which wasn't expelling much from the bowel because he was eating less solid food. We didn't understand the need for the antihistamine and repeatedly checked the drug bottles and the name on each label. We called Cathy at her office and explained what we felt was a mistake. She told us not to give Dad anything until we had called and cleared up the confusion to our satisfaction. If necessary, Dr Bell would go to our place to help us. We decided Dad must have received somebody else's prescriptions as well as his own. Both the doctor and the head nurse had signed off on the medication before he left the hospital and still a mistake had been made.

Just as Gail was about to phone the hospital the phone rang. A nurse from Dad's floor asked if we had given Dad any of the medicine. There had been a terrible mistake and if we had given some of those medicines to Dad he would have died. Gail spent some time with the caller sorting through what was his and what wasn't his and when he was to take which drug. Finally, she asked for the caller's name and wrote it down in our journal. Mistakes like this should not happen. True, Dad was terminal and his life expectancy had been reduced to a couple of weeks but ending his life with a mistaken drug being administered wasn't right. We were all angry such a mistake could happen and relieved we had the presence of mind to not just blindly follow the pill bottle directions without asking questions first.

We also decided Dad's dignity and modesty would be preserved for as long as we possibly could. His daughters would not be present when he went to the bathroom if it was at all possible. Ron and Steve and Mom would be able to take care of that detail. We also knew we would need to take shifts to help Dad change positions throughout the night or to get him pain medication or a drink of water. I said I'd take the first night shift. I needed to spend time with Dad. I wanted it to be just him and me.

# Monday, November 14, 2006

Subject: Good morning, Patty
Date:    2005 Nov 14—9:37
From:  Susan Arnold
To:      Village of South River

I hope you had a good weekend.

I'm sending under a separate e-mail a letter to the Personnel Committee informing them officially of my leave. Would you mind printing it off and putting a copy into Jim's mailbox for this evening's council meeting? Thanks.

How are things going?

Things here aren't great. The cancer is now in Dad's bones and other organs including his brain. He was released from the hospital on Friday and we have a hospital room set up here for him as we feel we can give him as good (and hopefully better) care here then in the hospital. We are currently doing shifts so he has someone available to move him or assist him throughout the twenty-four hour day. Enjoy your dad, Patty, no person should have to go through this hell at the end of a happy, productive life. Dad doesn't eat anything and only takes a bit of water which, apparently, is normal at this stage. It's heartbreaking but, he knows we are here and this seems to provide him with some comfort. He sleeps most of the time.

Ron went home yesterday to see the boys and check on the store and to visit his dad but will be back on Tuesday. Steve has taken this week off work as well so we have lots of support. Dad has had many visitors and phone calls. People in this community have been so concerned and want to help but there really isn't anything they can do. Just knowing they care is a great comfort to us. We've posted a sign limiting visits to five minutes. Dad will fall asleep but it is exhausting for him to make conversation at all but he tries valiantly.

I'd better go for now. I'll be in touch from time to time but, please, send me a note from the outside world. I miss you and want to hear about things in your life.

Again, if you have any questions just ask and I'll do my best to help or provide some guidance. Have a good day.

Love Susan


Today is Gail and Ron's birthday.

Ron went home to South River yesterday and will return tomorrow. Gail had a doctor's appointment in Kingston and she needed to pick up some personal things from her house. She arrived home in time for dinner.

Cathy and Steve brought some food to Mom and Dad's so we could all eat together. Mom and Dad gave Gail her birthday card and it was an extremely tearful time. Dad is becoming increasingly disoriented. He hasn't eaten since Sunday. Ron had gotten Dad to eat a few spoonfuls of pudding then but he hasn't eaten anything since. I don't think I'll ever be able to look at those little banana puddings without thinking of Dad.

I stayed up with Dad Friday night. He was so tired he didn't move much and whenever he did he seemed to think he was still at the hospital. We think he thought I was a nurse because every time I went near him he'd tell me to get away and yet, in the daylight, he knew it was me.

He is slipping further away from us.

The stream of visitors has been constant and we have now reached the point where a sign has been placed on the door asking friends to limit their visits to five minutes as the visits exhaust Dad quickly. Soon we will stop the visits. Dad would want to be remembered by his friends and neighbours as the active, vital man he has always been.

## Wednesday, November 16, 2005

**Dad** is still very much the centre of our family. We start everyday by visiting with him to see how his night had been and to ask if he needed anything. All day long we sit with him and talk quietly or we hold his hand and let him rest. He has a metal trapeze which hangs above his head which he uses for exercise. His right arm seems to have lost mobility because of the tumor under his shoulder bone but he continues to raise his left arm and grasp the bar. He can't pull himself up as his muscles have weakened to almost nothing but he likes to stretch his good arm as much as possible. The metal bar is also the source of much laughter. Without fail, anyone who is on the left side of Dad's bed will bump their head on the bar when they are helping to move him. Dad will look up at the latest victim with his blue eyes shining with amusement and he'll have a look on his face that says it all! We'll break into laughter because we never seem to learn to duck! One of Dad's medicines has a horrible taste. One night, when he knew it was time for that particular drug, he pretended to be asleep. When Cathy put down the medicine he opened his eyes and smiled at me! It amazes me that we find any amusement in this situation and, in truth, we are making many good memories. Surprisingly, it isn't all tears. Dad is primarily responsible for these good times. The rest of us take our cue from him. He loves to have all of us sitting around the bed talking about normal everyday things and, sometimes, he will contribute a thought or a memory to the conversation. He is very aware of what is going on around him and the routine of the household. We have made a point of not discussing his impending death or any funeral arrangements in front of him, even if he appears to be sleeping, because he may just be resting his eyes.

Despite the laughter there are also moments of intense pain and tears. Each one of us have experienced these times of despair. How quickly we are progressing to the end of this journey and the visible decline of Dad's health which we can measure on a daily basis. Sometimes I'm convinced I just can't do this. I just can't watch my father die. The pain of knowing it won't be long is almost physical. Sometimes I want to run away and wait for it to be over but then I'd never forgive myself for not being there for Dad. Most times I'm not thinking about my own pain. Most times I'm thinking about Dad's current needs. What can I do to help him now? I think all of us have put our own feelings on the back burner to concentrate on Dad. We'll have plenty of time in the future to deal with how we feel but the hopelessness and the tears do, sometimes, spill out now.

Dad's legs and feet have been giving him problems. We have been moving them for him and rubbing lotion into them to get the circulation going. Sometimes his feet are so hot he says they feel as though they are on fire and other times they feel ice cold.

We keep the livingroom drapes closed because the daylight hurts Dad's eyes. Motion and voices seem to overwhelm his senses so we speak in hushed tones and tell him what we are going to do before we do it.

"Dad, we're going to move you up in the bed. We'll count three and move you up a little and then we'll rest for a minute and when you're ready we'll move you up the rest of the way. Are you ready?" Then, in between the moves we will caress his forehead or his arms to soothe his nerves. We never act without telling him what is happening or asking his permission. He is still his own person and we respect his feelings and his requests. We are so careful not to talk as though he isn't in the room or not capable of understanding. Dad is still very much in control of his life. We are his assistances.

## Saturday, November 19, 2005

*The* home care nurses and the doctors are in to see Dad every day. They always say as they are leaving, "If you need us through the night don't hesitate to call." I'm starting to get really worried and a lot scared. I have never been with anyone at their death. Will I know when it is about to happen? What can I expect? Will there be a struggle? Gasping for air? What is the Death Rattle?

I finally got up the courage to ask one of the nurses to sit down at the kitchen table and explain to us what will happen.

She told us Dad will become extremely restless and he'll move his hands and feet more then normal for about a day before his passing. His breathing will become shallow and quick. He may have a day when he seems to improve. He won't want anything in his system. His body is shutting down. She promised to bring us a fact sheet the next day so we can read a little more and have a general idea of what to expect.

## Sunday, November 20, 2005

*Dad* can no longer swallow without great difficulty. We keep his lips moistened with a tongue sponge. He doesn't like the mint flavored ones. He wants only the plain ones.

We asked the doctor to prescribe a liquid painkiller to replace the pills which he just can't swallow without choking. We've been using a syringe (without the needle) to squirt the medicine into his mouth alongside his cheek so it will gently run down his throat. This seems to work much better and relieves the stress for him when he requires something to keep him comfortable. The doctor has left us some syringes for Cathy to administer morphine when/if the pain becomes worse, as it usually does at the end. He has refused the medicine which prevents the brain from swelling. He seems to not be bothered by much pain at all. He is barely taking anything for pain compared to what he could be given. As long as he remains peaceful and aware then we are grateful and we won't try to give him anything more then he requires.

Rob's dad is very low.

My arthritis has been flaring-up. My feet are so sore I can barely walk. Also, I have developed a blister-like rash on the palm of my hands. Both, I'm certain, are stress-related. The pharmacy has given me a cream to take away the itch and soothe the rash.

The minister has been in to visit Dad and sit with us several times this week. She has counted Dad and Mom as dear friends since her arrival in Sharbot Lake. Dad's illness has been difficult on her, too. She told us about the last church board meeting Dad chaired which was the week before his surgery in June. He hadn't said anything to the community yet and the minister had just announced she would be having her gallbladder removed that week. Apparently Dad expressed great concern over her upcoming surgery and was very fatherly and comforting as they discussed it. She had no idea what he was facing and will always remember his great compassion for the people around him and his ability to not dwell on his own troubles.

After one of her stories regarding Dad I felt myself tearing up and quietly left the family room to attend to something on the stove in the kitchen. I thought I'd made a quiet, natural exit but she was not fooled. She followed me into the kitchen and said, "You know, Susan, you don't always have to be the strong one. It's OK to cry". She gathered me into her arms and hugged me as if to pass along some of her strength and comfort. I must be a good actress because I certainly don't feel like I'm being very strong. I feel hollow and empty and easily crushed. Dad's tremendous strength makes any that I have seem insignificant in comparison. I'm overwhelmed by his poise and his concern for each of us.

Gail and Ron both have a sore neck and take turns using the heated oat bag to relax the muscles.

*Brandon*

*Every day Mom and Dad would call us and Uncle Steve would stay with us at night and make sure we went to school. I can remember one night hearing the phone ring and my Uncle Steve answering it. It was Mom. He talked to her for a while and I came into the room. He quickly got up and left the room so I couldn't hear the conversation. I knew Grandpa was getting worse.*

*For almost two weeks Mom and Dad and the rest of the family took care of Grandpa at their home in Sharbot Lake. It must have been hard for them.*

# Monday, November 21, 2005

---

Subject: Good Morning, Patty
Date:    2005 Mon 21—10:42
From:    Susan Arnold
To:      Village of South River

So nice to hear from both of you. Thank you for your e-mails and for your phone call, Patty. You have no idea how much they mean to me.

I hope you had a good weekend.

Life here has become torturous. I'm starting to hate the wall clock as it ticks away the hours of my father's life. The house is hushed and very somber. The laughter we had, even just a few days ago, is gone.

The people in the community have been wonderful. Someone drops by with a meal, a casserole or a plate of "goodies" everyday. Phone calls are still plentiful and offers to help are endless but there is really nothing to do but wait. One of the churches lit a candle for Dad on Saturday evening. I have represented our family the past two Sunday's by attending our regular Sunday service. The church has been a large part of my parent's life and I feel the need to uphold their traditions. Everywhere we go people want to know about Dad. Many approach with tears in their eyes. As I watch Dad lying so peacefully in his bed I'm truly amazed at the effect he has had on so many. I'm sure he'd be overwhelmed and very humbled to know the outpouring of concern he and our family have had showered on us.

Ron went home on Saturday and returned on Sunday. The boys seem to be coping well.

Patty, would you mind doing something for me? There is a poem hanging in my office entitled "Success". Would you

please courier it to me? I would like it to be read at the
funeral. The poem has always reminded me of Dad.

Thank you for your help and support and for your prayers.
Dad is not suffering and that's what I've been praying for;
as well as strength to get through this nightmare. I think
of you often.

Love Susan


We are exhausted. We have begun three people doing the night
shift. Dad as no mobility and two are needed to turn Dad and the
third is available in case an extra hand is required. Mom gets some
sleep upstairs but she will come down the stairs a couple of times
every night to check on Dad and see for herself how he is.

Cathy has left work for the week and feels the time is drawing near
for Dad to leave us. She and her family have moved into Mom and
Dad's, too.

When I lay in the family room at night listening to Dad's breathing
on the intercom it is hard to believe soon I'll never hear that sound
again. His breathing has always been loud and steady and it is a
sound I equate with security, comfort and home. His breathing
sounds so normal. How can this be happening?

Dad has been so patient. He never cries or becomes depressed. His
speech is almost gone. He was always a communicator and he still
manages to get his point across. When he needs to have his position
changed he gives us rudimentary directions and we try to follow.
When we are on the right track he will say "It's come'n". When we
are successful he'll say "Good" and when we're way off he'll say
"No". Ron and Gail are really so good with him. They seem to

know instinctively what he needs and are so comforting and gentle with him. Cathy and Steve work well together, too. Cathy, being a nurse, tells Steve what needs to be done and he helps make it happen. All I seem to be able to do is keep the kitchen organized, send out Thank You notes and hold Dad's hand. I feel so helpless although I feel as though my role is to support the others and to begin the task of making some arrangements and notifying some individuals of the nearness of Dad's departure.

Dad, while appearing to be asleep, is really very aware of the household routines and what is going on around him. This afternoon, one of Mom's sisters came for a visit and we all sat around Dad's bed telling stories from the past. We looked at Dad and saw a huge smile on his face! He understood everything we were saying and was enjoying the conversation. In truth, it wasn't any different then a hundred other conversations we'd had. We always sit around joking and reminiscing and Dad always enjoys these times together. Steve was talking about his logging and the fact the mill had closed and, although he had signed a contract with someone to harvest the logs he wondered what he should do. Dad, an hour after the conversation took place, managed to say, "Stick with the original contract." Even on his deathbed he is still helping us.

He doesn't seem to be experiencing any pain. His face is serene as we continue to administer a small amount of liquid Tylenol with codeine every four hours. So far, the morphine injections the doctor has left have not been necessary. I hope his pain management remains this simple for his sake and ours.

Last evening, as we were sitting with Dad, he reached into his mouth and took out his dentures and placed them on the table. He didn't say anything but the action almost seemed to say, "I'm not going to be using these anymore." His gums had shrunk inside his mouth and his dentures didn't fit and they must have felt uncomfortable to him. Dad was never seen without his dentures.

Dad's hands are very fidgety. He is moving them around a great deal today.

## Tuesday, November 22, 2005

---

Subject: Thanks, Patty!
Date:     2005, Nov 22—17:22
From:   Susan Arnold
To:       Village of South River

My package arrived. Thank you!

Dad is getting weaker and according to the professionals we don't have much time. Bitter sweet, eh? The minister has been with us quite a bit the past couple of days. She pulled me aside one day and told me I didn't have to always try to be the strong one just because I'm the oldest. Funny, I don't feel strong. I feel very weak and I seem to constantly be turning to Ron for strength. Perhaps on the outside I look strong but on the inside I'm a mess.

I'm glad things are going OK for you there. I'm glad I have you filling in for me. Don't stress too much. Unfortunately, I'll be back soon.

I'll let you know when something happens. The night times are the worst. When I'm on the night shift I can see what is happening but when I'm upstairs in my room the silence is ominous. In my lifetime, so far, this has been the hardest thing I've ever had to do. I pray you don't have to experience this.

Love Susan

# Wednesday, November 23, 2005, 6:25am

Dad is gone.

Cathy and Steve called us downstairs around 6:00am this morning. The time had arrived for us to say good-bye. Dad told Cathy to "Get Mom." His breathing was shallow but not raspy. His eyes were closed but I know he was aware of us. Mom held his hand. We gathered around him, tears streaming down our faces, and told him how much we loved him and we promised him we would take care of each other and we would remain a family and then, he was gone. No struggle. He simply stopped breathing. One second he was with us and the next there was only the hum of the oxygen machine and the sound of our sobbing.

I don't think I'll ever fear the end of life. Dad showed us how peaceful it can be. I can just hear him saying there is a time for everything. For us, it is the time for Dad to take one road and for us to continue our journey on another. His love and the memory of his devotion will travel with us until our two roads meet again.

I can't even think beyond this moment.

---

**Subject: Dad**
**Date:     2005, Nov 23—9:38**
**From:   Susan Arnold**
**To:        Village of South River**
**Dad passed away peacefully this morning at 6:25 with his family around him. Details have yet to be confirmed and I will let you know when I do. Ron is returning to South River this afternoon to be there to tell our boys. We didn't think it was right they should be told without one of us**

with them. Nothing else for now. My brain is pretty much mush. I'll be in touch.

Love Susan

*Brandon*

*Then one day after school Dad came home. As soon as he walked in the door he told us the roads were good. And then he said, "Grandpa died last night". I guess it was hard for him to tell us so he just said it. Our suits were hanging up in our rooms; we just hadn't seen them yet. Our aunt and uncle had gotten them ready for us. I just sort of sat down and watched TV because I didn't want to think about it. It kind of took awhile to process what had happened because it seemed so surreal.*

*I don't even remember the five and a half hour car ride there the next day. I was thinking what was going to happen when we came through the door. Would everyone be crying? Or would it be like any other time we came there?*

*When we got there we gave everyone our hugs and sat down in the livingroom with Mom. There was an awkward silence for the first fifteen minutes and then I think I saw Grandma crying which started a chain reaction throughout the house.*

*The next few days are a blur of tissues, faces of people we didn't know and places we didn't want to be.*

*Grandpa was brave and strong so we did the same for him. At least we tried.*

# Afterword

*Eighteen* months have passed since Dad died. Our family is gradually getting back on our feet and moving on with life. Each of us went through the grieving process in our own way; there really isn't a right or a wrong way to grieve. Some of us cried until we had no more tears, some of us withdrew into ourselves, some of us didn't talk about Dad or his illness, some of us talked about it for hours. A few of us took on so much work we'd be exhausted at night and some of us went to a doctor to discuss the physical aspects of grieving. One by one we are all emerging with renewed strength and have found joy in the people and places around us.

As fate would have it Rob's dad passed away a week after Dad. Both he and Gail have had to experience the painful emotions of the loss of two fathers at the same time.

Immediately after Dad's passing, and for the first few weeks, we all discovered we felt very transparent. As if all of our thoughts and emotions and the events of the past seven months were visible to everyone. I also felt as though I was re-emerging into the world. My own world had shrunk to the size of the livingroom where Dad's hospital bed had been. Many times I felt tentative and shaky; like a child learning to walk. Gradually, that feeling began to fade and we learned how to take control of our lives once again.

At first, my only memories of Dad were of him lying in his hospital bed. I relived the last two weeks of his life in vivid detail. I would remember every wrinkle, mark and bump on his face, arms and hands like a video which continuously played. I would recall each conversation and visitor he had until he could no longer speak. I was so afraid these memories, because they were etched so deeply in my mind, would be the only memories I would have of Dad. Once again, gradually, other memories from happier times came forward. Now, I can hear what he would have said in the many situations I have found myself in since his passing. I feel him with me and I carry him in my heart but the extreme sadness I also carried has gone.

The first year following Dad's death seemed to be a replay of the previous year. Dates on the calendar would explode like landmines. The anniversary of being told about his cancer, the anniversary of his surgery, the first chemotherapy treatment, his good days as well as his bad days were all dates on the calendar that marked the path we had just traveled. There are always the "first" this or that. Special occasions that have to be observed and rituals practiced by simply going through the motions as if we were being propelled by autopilot. Christmas and Dad's birthday passed a month after his funeral while we were still in a state of, what I now call, post-cancer trauma. We commemorated what would have been Mom and Dad's fiftieth wedding anniversary with a family weekend at our cottage and a lapel pin we had made for Mom. We decided we can't pretend these dates don't exist and so we try to meet them head on. It is difficult, but we have felt so proud of ourselves each time we have survived another landmine and I think, to some degree, we are each doing the best we can for each other and for Dad.

Before we knew it the first anniversary of his passing was upon us. My sisters, niece and Mom organized a slumber party, gave each other facials and had a chocolate tasting. On the actual anniversary we visited Dad's grave together. Dad loved when we got together and we felt it was appropriate for us to plan something which made the somber anniversary more a celebration of life. It was time to celebrate! We had survived the first year. There was, for me, almost a sense of relief which gave me permission to start enjoying life and participating in it fully once again.

Our family has had other reasons to celebrate over the past eighteen months. Job promotions have been earned, Bradley got his drivers license and Greg has his learners permit. Lindsay has successfully completed her first year at Queen's University. Cathy has been working hard on her university courses and doing very well. Steve's parents are about to celebrate their sixtieth wedding anniversary. Gail and Rob are building a new home, Brandon and I have been working on this book and Ron went to Chicago last summer with some friends to attend a major league ball game. In February of 2007, the Clark family travelled to Cancun, Mexico for a family vacation; the first without Dad. The trip was hard. Dad's enthusiasm and sense of fun was absent. The harder we tried to ignore the void that we all felt, the bigger the void seemed to grow. Life would never be the same but we were bravely stepping into the world on our own. Dad would approve.

Mom has been amazing. She misses Dad greatly but is carrying on. She has a brave face she puts on for the public and keeps her sadness hidden until she is alone. Mom makes herself attend community events and loves family gatherings. She doesn't sit at home feeling sorry for herself and finds something positive in everyday. Mom keeps busy and stays to a routine she is comfortable with. In March, Mom became the proud owner of, Kitty, a Blue Lynx Mitted-Ragdoll kitten that has found her way into Mom's heart, and ours. We're all so proud of Mom. She inspires us.

Looking back, I can see how each of us has grown in ways we didn't even consider possible. Our views on life, faith and the process of living have changed. We have redefined what our priorities are and place more emphasis on our own legacy. A healthy work ethic must be balanced with playtime. Dad used to tell us that and now we understand what he meant. I accept what I can't change and decide what I can change. I'm more tolerant and give people more consideration for the things they are going through which I may not know about. I say "I love you" more and try to eliminate the need for the words "would, could, should". We try to take life a little slower and take time to enjoy the moment we are in more often. We all have changed and I believe we are all much stronger. The healing takes time and everyone heals differently. But, we do heal and that is one of the miracles of being alive.

Honouring Dad will be easy; we just have to live life with purpose. To learn, appreciate, grow, be charitable and understand every journey has a beginning and an end. In between the start and the finish there will be many bumps on the road. How we handle those bumps will, ultimately, determine whether our journey is rewarding or if we discover, too late, how precious and wonderful life and living truly is.

# Part Five

# Conclusions

# Conclusions

***The*** original reason for this journal, as you know, was a way for me to express my feelings and help me cope during Dad's illness. Now, I find it interesting to see the many small, practical lessons we learned about taking care of ourselves and of Dad. I pray you are reading this book only out of interest and not because you are hoping to find useful information to help you and your family get over your own bump in the road. If that is your reason for reading this book, I give you my heart felt sympathies and a promise that you will find a way through this terrible time. I have listed below, in summary form, some of the many things we learned. I hope they help.

- We will be shocked and numb when we first get such news. Our head, our heart and our emotions all have to accept the diagnosis and they don't all accept at the same time. Listen to your body to hear what it needs you to do to help.

- Get a second opinion.

- Become informed about the specific cancer your family is dealing with. Learn the terminology and the procedures of treatment.

- When visiting a doctor's office it is helpful to have a family member (or close friend) accompany the patient. Moral support is important and so is the extra set of ears listening to the doctor. Take notes. It is amazing how much we don't really hear during an office visit and how quickly we forget when we leave the appointment. Short notes help to refresh everyone's memory and answer questions which might come up an hour afterward.

- Write down questions you don't find an answer for and take them to the patient's next appointment.

- Use your own judgment; don't blindly accept everything you are told. Ask questions.

- At the risk of being blunt: cancer patients are also research projects. Some of what doctors learn today may help you or another member of your family tomorrow. However, remind the doctors your family member is not a lab specimen and make sure he/she is given the opportunity to express how much experimentation they wish to have done on their body. Experimentation can adversely change their quality of life. This is when the "quality verses quantity" issue needs to be examined.

- The patient is often more calm than the family and friends but the patient still feeds off our positive energy and love.

- The cancer journey is really an emotional roller coaster and you will be filled with hope and despair, fear and relief, tears and laughter and the ride itself is exhausting. Hang on and every now and then give yourself permission to step off.

- Don't be afraid to discuss what you fear or to display your emotions to someone you trust. Sometimes your emotions may be anger at the situation or you might resent what you see as unfair. These feelings are normal so vent and don't feel guilty. The emotional cocktail swirling around inside you can't be stopped so you have to learn how to get these feelings out. In my case, besides talking, I kept this journal.

- Sometimes the patient needs to talk so be an active listener regardless of how uncomfortable you are with the chosen topic.

- Make an effort to keep to your regular routine. There is comfort in routine even if your mind is a jumble of thoughts.

- Attempt to look after your own health. Stress can weaken your immune system. Rest, food, exercise, fresh air and relaxation are all important when the patient is counting on you being there for them.

- Try to talk about other things some of the time. Our brain needs a break from the cancer and doctor talk.

- Your world will begin to revolve around appointment dates, amount of food eaten, quality of sleep and ways to bring comfort to your family member. Your moods may reflect how the patient is feeling; a good day for them means a good day for you.

- Don't feel guilty if you have to return to your own life some of the time. Unfortunately, the world doesn't stop because we need it to.

- Specialists tend to focus on the "main event" and discount the entire body of the patient. We found this most notably when Dad's shoulder, which hadn't been sore before the surgery, became sore immediately afterward. It was explained as having been over extended during the surgery and the position he was lying in during surgery. The explanation was reasonable. However, by September his shoulder still ached and it was still being explained as a result of the surgery. When we asked how this was possible when the surgery took place in June they decided it must be arthritis. In fact, he had a tumor growing underneath his shoulder girdle which was diagnosed in October. Don't let the doctors get tunnel vision.

- Patients on the surgical ward are treated very well. Unfortunately, when a patient is moved to the palliative ward or has "Do Not Resuscitate" on their chart then the care may become noticeably different.

- Sometimes patients become invisible and are spoken *about* instead of *to*.

- Patients quite often have a really good day the day after surgery, but the second day is much different.

- Things change quickly. A period of stable health can change instantly to a downward spiral and a downward spiral can reverse unexpectedly. Or, a patient can be retching one minute and eating dinner the next. Expect the unexpected.

- Your concept of what's "normal" will change constantly. Be prepared to adapt.

- Keep a notebook while your patient is in the hospital of what is prescribed, what doctor has been in and when, the time the last medication was given and anything else you feel appropriate in your situation.

- Doctors don't always have the best bedside manner. It can be upsetting when the doctor is being brutally honest. They deal with facts and their job is to give the patient this information. Your job is to give the patient comfort and love.

- Continue the notebook at home. This may help the doctors later.

- If the patient is tired don't be afraid to tell visitors rest is needed for your family member.

- Allow the patient to remain in control. Ask permission or ask if they'd like something. Don't just assume and proceed to do whatever you were planning to do. After all, they have cancer; they didn't stop being an individual.

- There are times when you will need to be creative. Trust yourself. I became a back support for Dad when he was sitting up in the bed to eat his dinner.

- A patient may appear to be sleeping but their muscles are deteriorating so their eye lids may just be closed. Be careful what you say; their hearing might be just fine.

- Move and speak slower. The ability to process words and actions slows down as the disease progresses.

- A patient may become sensitive to daylight and background noise as the body begins to shutdown.

- A patient may, as the disease progresses, experience personality changes.

- If it is possible, try to find a way to allow your loved one to spend the rest of their days in a loving home environment; surrounded by the people and things they hold dear. I believe the final gift we were able to give our dad was the time we spent at home, together, before his passing. We could pamper him and take care of him and show him, by simply holding his hand well into the night, how much he was loved. We showed him it was a privilege to have the chance to do for him just as he did for us all our lives.

- Stress and close, constant proximity can cause tension and strain between family members. It is not nice but it is normal. Recognize it for what it is and get over it. This is not the time to make more problems. Everyone is working for the same purpose; to make life more comfortable for the patient and to support each family member.

- Deal with practical matters before you need to. Pretending things aren't as bad as they are won't make the cancer go away. Ask questions.

- Don't just come in and take over. People become territorial about what they are doing because everyone feels so helpless and needs to feel needed. Find a job, something you can be responsible for: perhaps cleaning the bathroom or watering the plants.

- Keep track of kind gestures and gifts. A list will come in handy when you are sending out thank you notes.

- You may find it difficult to concentrate. My brain couldn't handle much in the way of a movie storyline or reading anything longer than a magazine article. Easy cross words, hand work, or "busy work" such as cleaning out a drawer or weeding a garden may help you focus long enough to give yourself a mental break from the stress.

- Learn how to lift properly so you don't throw out your back.

- Lots of hugs. I was amazed at how much strength we could get from one little hug. Make this time a very special time in your family's history.

- Try to keep a sense of humor. Your family member shouldn't leave this world without experiencing as much joy and laughter as possible.

- Tell your family member how much you love them and remind them of things you did together in the past. Knowing they have been a positive impact in your life is very important.

- Mend fences. We want our loved one to rest in peace and we want to continue on without regrets. Our family was lucky and didn't have to spend precious time mending fences but not everyone is as fortunate. Regardless of what the nature of the problem was in the past, the sad truth is, it doesn't matter any more. We only get one chance to do this right.

- Regardless of how prepared we think we are for our family member's passing or how long we've had to accept the news; it is still a shock.

- Look for blessings where you can find them; a beautiful sunset, a great cup of coffee, a card of support, a visit from a neighbor, a chance to spend time with people you care about, etc

- This journey changes everyone. Don't judge too harshly when the people around you don't react the way you expect them to react. They have changed, too, and many of us don't recognize the change until later.

- Support one another. This is a difficult time for everyone and we each need different things to help us get through this bump in the road.

- You will get through this painful time. As hard as it is to imagine now, you will be happy again. Time really does heal our wounds. Time will never take away our memories or the special place in our heart where each of our loved-ones live, but it will take away the sharp pain of separation and the flat, two-dimensional world around us. There will be a day when you will begin to look forward more than you look behind. I promise.

- The length of time and the way you grieve shouldn't be defined by somebody else. Do what is right and comfortable for you.

Thank you for taking the time to get to know a little about my family and our journey with cancer. My father played a very important part in making this time meaningful to our family and we consider ourselves very fortunate to have had his guidance to the very end and his example of living life with purpose and meaning to help get us back on track after he was gone.

Unfortunately, our family is not alone. Every year many families, perhaps yours, hit their very own bump in the road. Your experience will be unique and special but some of the lessons my family learned may help you to know a little more about what lies ahead of you. I hope our story will give you some comfort and reassure you that you will not only have strength, you'll have *incredible* strength, to navigate you and your family over this difficult bump in the road.

God bless.

# *About the Author*

Susan Arnold is the Clerk-Administrator for the Village of South River and lives in South River, Ontario with her husband, Ron, and their two boys, Greg and Brandon.

978-0-595-46040-3
0-595-46040-2